Eating Disorders in America

Recent Titles in the
CONTEMPORARY WORLD ISSUES
Series

Books in the **Contemporary World Issues** series address vital issues in today's society such as genetic engineering, pollution, and biodiversity. Written by professional writers, scholars, and nonacademic experts, these books are authoritative, clearly written, up-to-date, and objective. They provide a good starting point for research by high school and college students, scholars, and general readers as well as by legislators, businesspeople, activists, and others.

Each book, carefully organized and easy to use, contains an overview of the subject, a detailed chronology, biographical sketches, facts and data and/or documents and other primary source material, a forum of authoritative perspective essays, annotated lists of print and nonprint resources, and an index.

Readers of books in the Contemporary World Issues series will find the information they need in order to have a better understanding of the social, political, environmental, and economic issues facing the world today.

Eating Disorders in America

A REFERENCE HANDBOOK

David E. Newton

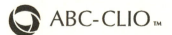

ABC-CLIO™

An Imprint of ABC-CLIO, LLC
Santa Barbara, California • Denver, Colorado

Library of Congress Cataloging-in-Publication Data

Names: Newton, David E., author.
Title: Eating disorders in America : a reference handbook / David E. Newton.
Description: Santa Barbara, California : ABC-CLIO, LLC, [2019] | Series: Contemporary world issues | Includes bibliographical references and index.
Identifiers: LCCN 2019000288 (print) | LCCN 2019001109 (ebook) | ISBN 9781440858604 (ebook) | ISBN 9781440858598 (print : alk. paper)
Subjects: | MESH: Feeding and Eating Disorders | United States
Classification: LCC RC552.E18 (ebook) | LCC RC552.E18 (print) | NLM WM 175 | DDC 362.19685/26—dc23
LC record available at https://lccn.loc.gov/2019000288

ISBN: 978-1-4408-5859-8 (print)
      978-1-4408-5860-4 (ebook)

23 22 21 20 19   1 2 3 4 5

This book is also available as an eBook.

ABC-CLIO
An Imprint of ABC-CLIO, LLC

ABC-CLIO, LLC
147 Castilian Drive
Santa Barbara, California 93117
www.abc-clio.com

This book is printed on acid-free paper ∞

Manufactured in the United States of America

Contents

Preface

Eating disorders are an issue of significant concern in the United States and many other parts of the world today. Although definitive statistics are not generally available, most estimates place the number of individuals with eating disorders to be about 1 percent. Although that number may seem small, in the United States it would mean that there are more than 3 million men and women, boys and girls, in the country with an eating disorder. That statistic also means that eating disorders are the most common of all mental health problems today. They are also the most common cause of death among all types of mental illness.

The cluster of conditions that are included in the rubric of *eating disorder* includes some disorders that have been known and studied for centuries, such as anorexia nervosa and bulimia nervosa. Other conditions now recognized as eating disorders are of more recent interest; some have not even been clearly defined for more than a few decades. The conditions known as other specified feeding or eating disorder (OSFED) and avoidant/restrictive food intake disorder (ARFID), both of which were first formally defined for the first time in the *Diagnostic and Statistical Manual of Mental Disorders-V (DSM-V)*, were released in 2013. Although still poorly understood, these two categories of eating disorders are now recognized as far more common than are the classical disorders of anorexia and bulimia.

Discussions of eating disorders may or may not include mention of overweight and obesity. Some experts prefer to reserve the latter term for the five categories of conditions mentioned in *DSM-V*—anorexia, bulimia, binge eating disorder, ARFID, and OSFED—while others choose to include overweight and obesity within this definition. In this book, the broader definition of eating disorders is adopted, although attention to overweight and obesity is somewhat abbreviated. The reason for this decision has been that a very significant body of literature now exists on overweight and obesity that is available to the general public and the researcher. Most of the discussion here, then, focuses on the aspects of eating disorders for which such resources may not be so readily available.

The first two chapters of the book are designed to provide a broad, general understanding of the nature of eating disorders; their characteristic features and the history of their appearance and study, primarily in Western civilization; risk factors and effects for each of the disorders; and a review of the prevention and treatment programs that have been developed to deal with eating disorders. Both chapters include extensive citations. The reason for these citations is not only, as usual, to provide the basis for remarks in the main text but also to make readers aware of the vast literature on the topics discussed here. After all, the book is intended as a reference handbook and resource guide for readers who would like to learn more about the topic or continue their own research on this subject. The chapter references are designed to assist in those objectives.

Remaining chapters of the book are included to further assist those objectives. Those chapters focus on books, articles, and electronic sources of further information on eating disorders; a relevant chronology of events in the field; a list of useful terms in understanding the subject of eating disorders; a selection of documents and data that provide additional information on past and recent history in the field of eating disorders; and an annotated list of important individuals and organizations in the field of eating disorders. Finally, a chapter on perspectives has provided individuals with an opportunity to write brief essays about their own experiences with, recent research on, or other topics related to the subject of eating disorders.

Eating Disorders in America

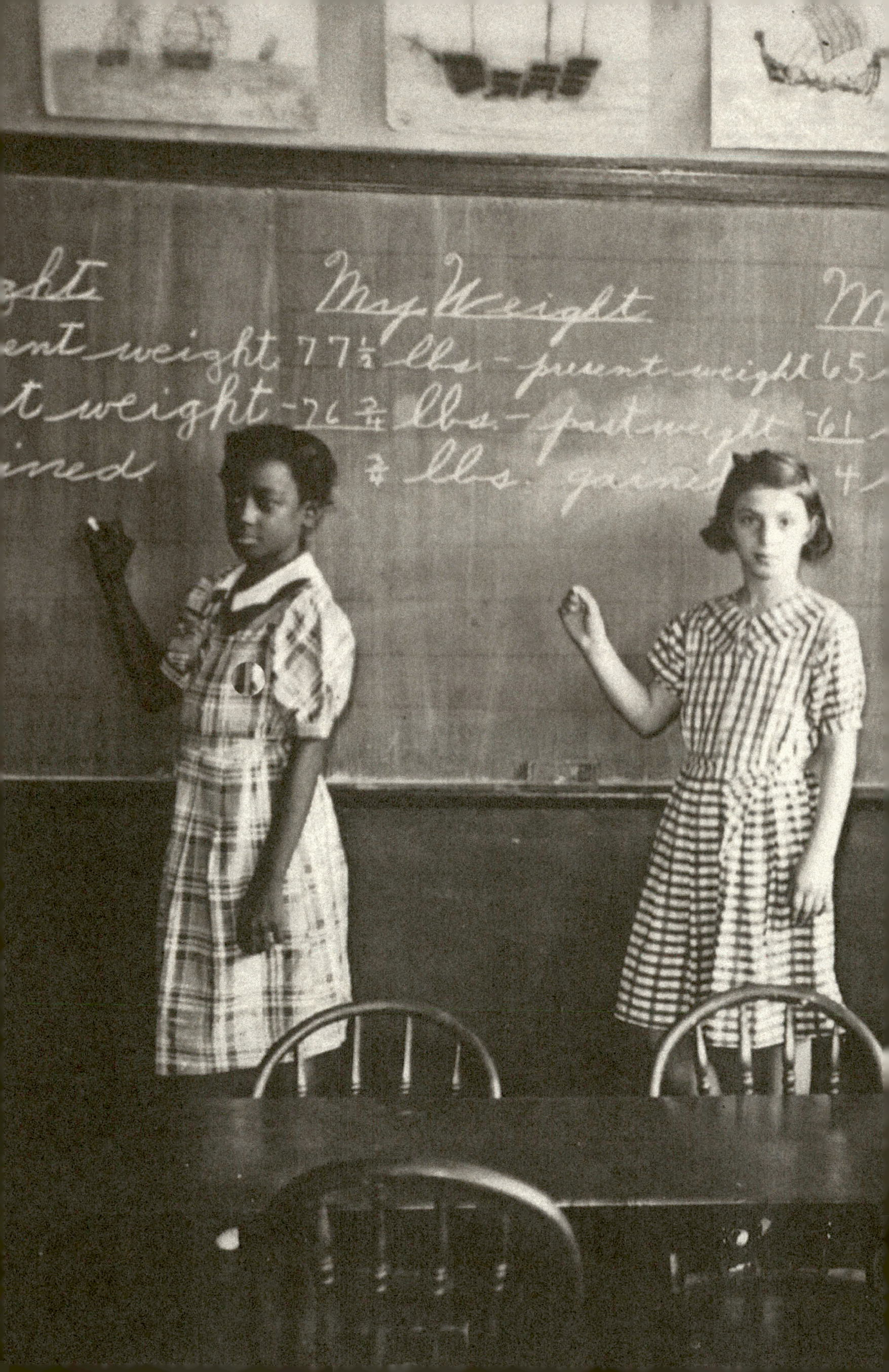
My Weight
weight 77½ lbs. - present weight 65
weight - 76¾ lbs. - past weight 61
¾ lbs. gained 4

What is it with Annette? She has changed so much over the past few months that I hardly recognize my long-time good friend. She's constantly staring at herself in the mirror, and she's started wearing the ugliest clothes, much too big for her and not at all flattering. And it's weird to be around her in the cafeteria. She won't even look at most of the foods we're served, and she takes only the smallest portions you can imagine. She says she's a vegan now . . . the same girl who used to gobble down hamburgs almost every day for lunch. Why, I even saw her at lunch turn her head and spit out the food she had been chewing. I think there's something wrong with Annette.

There is. Annette almost certainly has an eating disorder. An eating disorder is defined as any condition in which an individual follows an irregular pattern of eating, either eating less or more than one would or should normally eat. These eating patterns reflect a person's (usually incorrect) perception of his or her body characteristics, such as "I'm too fat" or "Parts of my body are too big or too large." In most cases, an eating disorder is a mental or emotional issue, not a malfunction of the body's biological functioning.

New Jersey school children determine changes in their weight by comparing past and present weights on the blackboard, ca. 1940–1950. (National Library of Medicine)

An Overview of Eating Disorders

Definitions

Perhaps the best-known eating disorders are bulimia, anorexia, and obesity. But other types of eating disorders have also been recognized. Among those eating disorders are the following:

- *Anorexia* (anorexia nervosa) is characterized by an extreme effort to avoid gaining weight by simply cutting back dramatically on the amount of food ingested.

- *Bulimia* (bulimia nervosa) is a condition in which a person consumes large amounts of food and then vomits or uses some other method to avoid gaining weight, processes that are known as *purging*.

- *Binge eating disorder* (*BED*) occurs when a person eats unusually large quantities of food that are *not* followed by purging. One consequence of BED is typically overweight and/or obesity.

- *Avoidant/restrictive food intake disorder* (*ARFID*) is a technical term used by psychiatrists, psychologists, nutritionists, and other experts in the field to describe a condition similar to anorexia, which does not also include negative feelings about one's body.

- *Other specified feeding and eating disorders* (*OSFED*) is a fairly new term used by professionals in the field to describe eating patterns that may resemble anorexia or bulimia but that differs in some important ways from those two conditions.

- *Orthorexia* (or orthorexia nervosa) is a condition in which a person is obsessed by eating only certain types of foods because they are thought to be the healthiest for one's body while strictly avoiding other foods that are thought to be harmful or unnecessary in one's diet.

- *Rumination disorder* is recognized as a condition in which a person vomits on a regular basis over a period of time (at least a month) with no known biological or anorexia- or bulimia-related cause.

- *Pica* is a term that refers to the ingestion of materials that are not normally thought of as any kind of food, such as paint chips, dirt, kitchen or cleaning products (e.g., baking soda or cornstarch), or cigarette butts or ashes.
- *Obesity* (and overweight) is a term that describes the condition that results when a person eats much more than is needed to live a normal, healthy life. Overweight and obesity may be caused by abnormal body functions or improper attitudes about one's body and/or lifestyle. (The list of eating disorders and criteria for their diagnosis can be found in the *Diagnostic and Statistical Manual of Mental Disorders-V* [*DSM-V*], American Psychiatric Association 2013, xxi, 329–354; all of these disorders will be discussed in more detail later in this chapter.)

Statistics

Statistics on the incidence and prevalence of eating disorders in the United States are difficult to come by, although some organizations have made estimates about these numbers. (*Incidence* means the number of new cases of a condition that appear within some time period, such as one year. *Prevalence* refers to the total number of individuals who have that condition during any given time period.) Based on studies conducted between 2007 and 2016, for example, the National Association of Anorexia Nervosa and Associated Disorders estimates that at least 30 million people in the United States suffer from an eating disorder at any one given time. Those eating disorders are responsible for the highest rate of mortality of any mental condition. Evidence suggests that eating disorders are common especially among women above the age of 30 (13 percent of all American women in that age group), transgender college students (16 percent), active military personnel (5.5 percent of women and 4 percent of men), and sexual minority college students (3.5 percent of women and 2.1 percent of men).

A 2012 comprehensive review of essentially all studies of the prevalence and incidence of eating disorders conducted around the world found incidence rates of anorexia nervosa ranging from 4.2 to 4.7 percent in the United Kingdom between 1994 and 2000; from 7.4 to 7.7 percent in the Netherlands between 1993 and 2000; and from 0.27 to 0.49 percent in Finland between 1990 and 1998. Similar data for the incidence of bulimia nervosa were about 0.2 percent in Finland between 1975 and 1979; from 6.1 to 8.6 percent in the Netherlands between 1985 and 1999; and from 6.6 to 12.2 percent in the United Kingdom between 1995 and 2000 (Smink, van Hoeken, and Hoek 2012).

Much more complete and recent data with regard to the incidence and prevalence of obesity in the Unites States are available. In its most recent report on the condition, the National Center for Health Statistics of the Centers for Disease Control and Prevention estimated that the overall rate of obesity in the United States between 2011 and 2014 was 36.5 percent. That rate varied widely, however, among various subgroups. It was higher for women (38.3 percent) than for men (32.3 percent); it was higher for older adults aged 40–59 (40.2 percent) and above the age of 60 (37.0 percent) than for younger adults aged 20–39 (32.3 percent); it was higher for blacks (48.1 percent) and Hispanics (42.5 percent) than for Caucasians (34.5 percent) and Asian Americans (11.7 percent); and it was higher for younger children (8.9 percent) than for young adults 20.5 percent). The trend for obesity in American adults has trended upward over the past two decades, from 30.5 percent in 1999 to 37.7 percent in 2014, and has remained relatively constant among children and young adults (13.9–17.2 percent) during the same period (Ogden et al. 2016).

Eating Disorders in History

Obesity

There have been discussions and debates throughout human history as to what the "ideal" human figure should look like. At times, societies have favored very heavy (usually) women, and at other times, the emphasis has been placed on a lithe figure. Probably no period illustrates this fact better than the Upper Paleolithic era, which lasted from about 50,000 BCE to about 10,000 BCE. Archaeologists have now discovered more than 200 figurines of grossly obese women that are collectively referred to as the *Venus figurines*. These statues have been recovered from nearly every part of Europe and eastward as far as Siberia. They are carved out of calcite, limestone, steatite, ivory, bone, and other materials. They depict very heavy women, individuals who would certainly be classified as obese and even grossly obese in today's world.

The first of these objects to have been discovered was found in about 1864 by the Marquis de Vibraye at Laugerie-Basse (Dordogne), France, during the excavation for a new building at the site. Vibraye called his discovery *La Venus impudique* (the immodest Venus), thought to be a contrast with a famous statue from ancient Greece, the *Venus Pudica* (the modest Venus), a representation of the goddess Aphrodite, who is covering her genital region with her hand (White 2006). The oldest of these figures, now known as the Venus of Hohle Fels, or the Venus of Schelklingen, has been dated to about 35,000–40,000 BCE. The figure was discovered in 2008 by Nicholas J. Conard, an archaeologist at the University of Tübingen, Germany. The woman depicted in the figurine has enormous breasts and hips and very large, explicit genitalia (Wilford 2009; for photographs of some of these figures, see Holloway 2014).

Trying to explain the purpose of such figurines has become something of a parlor game for archaeologists. There are essentially no concrete data to explain their (as we might term it today) bizarre physical features. This problem is especially difficult to solve because there is abundant archaeological evidence to indicate that the majority of men and women living during this period were muscular but slight. This finding makes sense when one reviews the stage of development at which these hunters and gatherers existed (Dixson and Dixson 2011; Józsa 2011). The most common hypotheses are that the women depicted were thought of as goddesses, to whom worship was directed; as fertility symbols, reminding people of the importance of becoming pregnant and bearing children; or as the ideal female form to which living women should strive to become. One rationale for the last of these suggestions is that very fat women (and men) are symbols of highly successful individuals in a society who are able to eat as much food as they want and who therefore become obese. In such a case, the figurines could be a prod to living women to strive for good marriages through which their husbands could supply all of their needs and desires and not concretely as the physical form that they should attain (Molnar 2011; Tripp and Schmidt 2013).

Obesity was also a prominent feature of ancient Egyptian culture. Evidence from the study of mummies and pictographs suggests that obesity was not uncommon, although apparently more to be found among the elite members of society than among commoners. Some examples include a doorkeeper in the temple of Amon-Ra Khor-en-Khonsu; a cook in the tomb of Ankh-ma-Hor; and a royal functionary, the well-known Sheikh al Balad (Bray and Bouchard 2014). One interesting discovery has been that existing depictions of famous Egyptian rulers and other members of the upper class do not necessarily conform with what archaeologists have learned about the same individuals from modern studies of their mummified remains. For example, statues of Queen Hatshepsut, who ruled from 1478 to 1458 BCE, generally show her as a slender, healthy individual. However, modern-day studies of her mummy have discovered that she was probably quite obese and afflicted with diabetes. One observer has concluded from such evidence that "the ancient Egyptians intuitively figured that thin and trim people were more attractive than obese ones and created their pictures accordingly" (Eades 2007).

The common theme that appears to run through much of both ancient and modern history, then, is something like, "obesity is a sign that someone has enough wealth and/or status to eat unlimited amounts of food, and moderate levels of obesity are probably acceptable, but excess (what scientists today would call *morbid*) obesity is not, because of the illnesses that seem to attend that condition." In ancient Greece, that theme continues in the work of some writers on medical topics. For example, probably the most famous of Greek physicians, Hippocrates (460–370 BCE), mentions the health problems associated with obesity and ways in which the problem can be treated. In the *Aphorisms*, for example, he notes that "persons who are naturally very fat are apt to die earlier than those who are slender" (Hippocrates 1868). He goes on to say that overeating is "injurious to the health" and then recommends that the best way to avoid problems associated with overweight is to exercise regularly (Bray and Bouchard 2014, 5; Christopoulou-Aletra and Papavramidou 2004, 513).

Many of Hippocrates's views toward obesity were carried over by ancient Roman physicians. Among the most important of these practitioners was Aelius (or Claudius) Galenus (130–210 CE), almost universally known today simply as Galen. Galen's views on obesity were particularly trenchant because of his later fame as a physician. For more than 1,000 years after his death, the most common medical practices were based on so-called Galenic medicine, a vast set of principles as to the causes of disease and methods for treating such diseases. The most basic principle of Galenic medicine was the dogma of the four humors—black bile, yellow bile, blood, and phlegm—whose balance or imbalance was deemed to be responsible for a person's health and well-being. An excess or deficiency of any one or more humors would be manifested by cancer, diabetes, or some other type of disease. In Galen's view, obesity was caused by an excess of blood in comparison with the other three humors (Papavramidou, Papavramidis, and Christopoulou-Aletra 2004). One method for treating overweight, then, was bleeding, a process for removing that excess blood from the body:

> The increase of Flesh is caused through plenty of good Blood, made by a temperate Liver out of meats of good juyce. . . . The increase of fat is caused by the oyliness and fattiness of the blood, falling out of the veins into the membranous parts, and there congealed . . .
>
> Signes are needless. The consequences thereof, are, an hindrance of the motions and operations of the body: also shortness of breath, by reason of the passages being stopt.
>
> For the Cure; first the Liver vein must be opened, from whence let a small quantity of blood be drawn.
>
> Secondly, the Patient must shun all such things as generate blood too plentifully, and use a very spare diet. (Galen 1662)

Galen recognized three general body types that exceeded that which was considered "normal" at the time. He called these three forms of overweight *pachis* (fat), *efsarkos* (chubby; from *ef* ["well"] and *sarka* ["flesh"]), and polysarkos (obese; from *poli* ["excess"] and *sarka*). The first two of these he regarded as relatively harmless, if not necessarily desirable. The third body type, however, was one that was likely to become associated with a variety of medical problems. In order to lose weight and avoid these problems, Galen recommended essentially the same approaches that experts on obesity suggest today: reduce one's intake of foods, choose foods that are healthy, and increase one's activities (Berryman 2012; Galenus and Siegel 1976).

Attitudes about obesity during the Middle Ages appear to have largely mirrored those of earlier times. During the period, survival was difficult for the vast majority of humans, and, as almost always, obesity represented an escape form the dull and deadly life of the less-well-off. Thus, many of the portraits and statues from the period show both men and women who are obviously well fed (and thus, by extension, successful and probably powerful). To many experts, these attitudes culminated in the work of the Flemish painter Peter Paul Rubens (1577–1640). Rubens, for all his other masterly work, is still probably best known for his depiction of robust and sometimes-nearly-obese women, a style that has come to be known as Rubenesque (Van Wyhe 2017).

Toward the end of the Renaissance period (late seventeenth century), attitudes with regard to obesity began to change in Europe. In his masterful book on the history of obesity (Vigarello 2013), French historian and sociologist Georges Vigarello points to two fundamental changes in societal attitudes about obesity. One change involved an increasingly negative view toward and about obese individuals. He turns to Shakespeare's Falstaff as the embodiment of the "accumulation of insults" directed at obese people. Among the many insults hurled at Falstaff by Prince Hal (Prince Henry, later to become King Henry V) is Hal's depiction of Falstaff as "this sanguine coward, this bed-presser, this horseback-breaker, this huge hill of flesh" (Shakespeare ca. 1597; Vigarello 2013, 47–48). No longer a model of wealth, success, and power, obese individuals had now become for many people the embodiment of an "oaf," worthy of ridicule and criticism. As another example of this attitude, Vigarello quotes an observer of the period, French magistrate François-Auguste de Thou, who ridicules certain women who must travel by carriage because "their overly large breasts prevent them from riding horseback" (Vigarello 2013, 24).

The second change to which Vigarello refers is an increasing attention to possible medical treatments for the description, cure, prevention, or other treatment of obesity. This change appears to come about as more scientific and medical evidence begins to appear, correlating obesity with a variety of discrete medical problems, such as apoplexy, dropsy, fatigue, gout, and respiratory problems (*apoplexy* refers to a sudden death resulting from some type of bleeding within the body, such as might occur during a stroke; *dropsy* is a term used to describe the accumulation of fluids within some part of the body, as might occur as the result of congestive heart failure) (Eknoyan 2006, 424). The treatments devised for obesity were not, however, based on any existing scientific evidence but reflected the medical profession's best guesses as to what might solve a person's problem of overweight. Since Galen's theory of the four humors still obtained in the medical world, one such "cure" was bloodletting, in the hope of removing the excess of blood thought to be the cause of the condition. Other treatments ranged from straightforward physical restraints on a person's body (corsets) to the use of methods for reducing food intake (dieting, purging, and the ingestion of noxious materials, such as vinegar, lemons, and chalk) to vigorous physical exercise (Vigarello 2013, 69–78).

By the end of the eighteenth century, a fundamental difference of opinion regarding the nature of obesity had developed. Some people, reflecting a long tradition of views on the subject, thought of the condition as a moral failure, an inability of obese people to have the strength to refrain from overeating; they were, in other words, fat because they had no self-control. And that self-control was seen as a conscious decision to behave in a way that was inappropriate and harmful to the body. Indeed, obesity was often specifically associated with at least two of the seven deadly sins defined by the early Christian church: sloth and gluttony. As an example, one individual who, himself, dealt with the challenge of obesity, the Scottish physician George Cheyne (1671–1743), wrote at one point that "to cut off our Days by Intemperance, Indiscretion, and guilty Passions, to live miserably for the sake of gratifying a sweet Tooth, or a brutal Itch; to die Martyrs to our Luxury and Wantonness, is equally beneath the Dignity of human Nature, and contrary to the Homage we owe to the Author of our Being" (Cheyne 1724, 4; also see Haslam and Haslam, 2009; Sawbridge and

Fitzgerald. 2009; Cheyne eventually switched to a vegetarian diet, lost weight, lived more than 70 years, and widely recommended his "cure" for obesity; the religious view of obesity as a moral issue—specifically, as a sin—remains a significant part of Christian teachings today; see, e.g., Ashley 2007; Maynard 2010; Merrill 2016; Tautges 2007).

This moralistic concern about obesity developed in sharp contrast to another perspective, namely, that obesity was a medical problem that could be understood and treated only by understanding the basic principles of chemistry, physics, anatomy, physiology, and other sciences. The first monograph that can be said to be devoted exclusively to the subject of obesity appeared in 1727 with the publication of English physician Thomas Short's book entitled *A Discourse Concerning the Causes and Effects of Corpulency* (Smart 1728). That publication was followed three decades later by a similar book by the Dutch physician Malcolm Flemyng (Flemyng 1757). Both of these books reflected the rise of a movement that began to think of obesity as a medical problem, not strictly a moral, social, or personal issue.

This new approach to the study of obesity came about as part of a much larger revolution, the rise of modern science. Beginning in the late seventeenth century and extending into the early nineteenth century, a number of fundamental discoveries were made in what we now think of as modern biology, chemistry, and physics, some of which had profound effects on the way in which some scholars viewed problems of obesity. The story of these changes, especially with respect to their influence on the study of obesity, is a long and complex one for which there are a number of excellent references but which will not be discussed in detail here (see, e.g., Bray and Bouchard 2014, 7–10, figures 1.2, 1.3, and 1.4; Eknoyan 2006; Fairburn and Brownell 2005, table 6.1 and chapter 69; McCaw 1917; Truswell 2013).

One example of the development of a "scientific" view of obesity may, however, be useful. This example is based on a basic change in the way in which scholars observed and studied nature. For nearly all of human civilization, descriptions of plants, animals, the human body, and other natural phenomena were *qualitative* in nature, that is, expressed in terms (in the case of obesity) such as *fat, gross, corpulent, lithe*, and *emaciated*. There was no effort to express these characteristics in *quantitative* terms, such as a specific height or weight.

But one of the basic precepts set out by the founders of modern science, such as the great Italian physicist Galileo Galilei, was that one could truly understand nature only when it was expressed in mathematical terms. Indeed, a slogan often heard even today is that "mathematics is the language of physics (or science)." As biology, chemistry, physics, and the other sciences developed, then, it became incumbent on researchers to measure phenomena, such as the speed of a falling object, the height of a column of mercury supported by atmospheric temperature, and the weight of an individual person. This requirement, in turn, created the necessity of inventing or developing instruments with which one could take precise measurements, such as the barometer and thermometer.

One can appreciate this change by examining the life of one important individual, Adolphe Quetelet, a Belgian polymath who made contributions in mathematics, statistics, astronomy, and sociology. From an early age, Quetelet was interested in using science to describe human characteristics and behavior. He spent much of his life in collecting data on every conceivable feature of men and women, such as their height, weight, circumference of the chest, length of the upper arm, and width of the foot. From these data, Quetelet then used statistics to calculate the "ideal" man and "ideal" woman, the individual in both cases who fell in the middle range of all his statistics.

These data led almost inevitably to a consideration of those who were not average, that is, those who were *statistically* heavier or lighter than the "ideal" individual. Quetelet determined that the best way to describe the range of body types about which he had gathered data was a measure that was originally called the *Quetelet index*, now better known today as the *body mass index* (*BMI*). This number is calculated by dividing a person's body mass (his or her weight) in kilograms by the square of his or her height (in meters). Thus a person who weighs 50 kilograms and stands 1.4 meters in height would have a BMI of $50 \div (1.4)^2 = 50 \div 1.96 = 25.5$.

As a result of Quetelet's research, then, it had become possible by the end of the eighteenth century to go beyond calling a person "fat" or "obese" or "skinny" and specify precisely "how fat," "how obese," or "how skinny" that person is. Beyond that, one could also decide what to call a person with any one of many possible BMI scores. That process has remained in use to the present day. Experts in the field of obesity have decided, for example, that anyone with a BMI of 18.5–24.9 is "normal." By contrast, anyone with a BMI of less than 18.5 is labeled as "underweight," while a person with a BMI of 25.0–29.9 is considered to be "overweight" and a BMI of over 29.9 is said to be "obese." Some individuals and organizations recognize a fifth category for those with a BMI above 39.9: morbidly obese. The condition reflected by this term generally describes a person who is so far overweight that carrying out the simple normal tasks of everyday life, such as walking and breathing, can become so serious that he or she is at risk of death. (To calculate your own BMI and learn more about the measure, see Body Mass Index 2015. For more information about Quetelet and the BMI, see Eknoyan 2008.)

Brief mention can be made of some of the other important events relating to the study of obesity in the nineteenth century:

- In 1826, French jurist and politician Anthelme Brillat-Savarin published his now-classic work, *The Physiology of Taste, or Transcendental Gastronomy*, considered to be the first book devoted entirely to eating, diet, obesity, weight loss, and related topics. His weight-loss diet is said to have become widely popular among individuals trying to lose weight

(Daley 2015; the text of the book is available online at *The Physiology of Taste* 1826/2004).

- In 1849, English physician Arthur Hassall reported on his study of discrete units ("vesicles" or "globules") found in children and adults responsible for the storage of fats in the human body, which, he says, "some deem to be true cells." The report appears to be the earliest possible description of the structure, composition, and changes in fat cells (Bray 1993b; Hassall 1849, 1851).

- In 1863 English undertaker William Banting published what is believed to be the first weight-loss booklet in the English language, entitled *Letter on Corpulence, Addressed to the Public*. The book summarized the dietary program Banting had followed to reduce his weight of 202 pounds in 1862 to 156 pounds about a year later. (Banting's height was about 5 feet, 5 inches.) Banting's contribution has been retained in the form of the term *banting*, once widely used and today less commonly so, meaning "to be on a diet" (Edwardes 2003; Groves 2003; the text of Banting's booklet can be found at Banting 1864).

- In 1896, American chemist W. O. Atwater and his colleagues described the construction and operation of a human calorimeter to measure the effects of exercise and nutrition on human metabolism and, hence, weight gain and loss. The device is used to measure the amount of heat produced (and thus energy released) by the human body within a sealed container by measuring temperature changes in water circulating through and around the chamber (Bray 1993a; Katch 1999; the first report on the device can be found at Atwater, Woods, and Benedict 1897).

During the twentieth century in the United States (and some other parts of the world), obesity was treated as a medical problem that can be studied and understood using a variety of tools from science and mathematics. Somewhat surprisingly perhaps, one of the strongest influences on this trend was the creation of professional societies of actuarial specialists in the late part of the eighteenth century and early part of the twentieth century. Most of these specialists were employed by insurance companies to estimate the risk of potential policyholders, a crucial factor in setting premium rates. Insurance companies became increasingly efficient at collecting data from their clients to determine the factors that affect death rates among those clients. They discovered early on that weight was one important factor, with heavier individuals being at significantly greater risk than were lighter individuals. At the 12th annual meeting of the Association of Life Insurance Medical Directors of America in 1901, for example, one speaker provided data showing that the death rate of those individuals who were classified as overweight was about 34 percent higher than it was for individuals with normal weight (Rogers 1901, 283). He also suggested that the risk of death increased with the degree to which a person was overweight.

In order to conduct and interpret data such as these, insurance companies had to establish some set of "normal," or "standard" values for weight. In this regard, they were carrying on the tradition that had begun with the work of Quetelet in trying to decide what a normal or standard weight was. During the first decade of the twentieth century, various life insurance companies developed and published a number of "standard tables of weight and height" that indicated the predicted life span of individuals based on those characteristics (Komaroff 2016; for an example of some of the earliest of such tables, see Fish 1867). The underlying message presented by these tables was expressed by one observer in 1909 when he noted that "overweight universally shortens life. Overweight is a burden, not a reserve fund" (as quoted in Bivins and Marland 2016). The basic foundation had been established for identifying the "standard" (or "recommended" or "best") weights for a person's given height that continues to the present day.

Still, issues of obesity in the United States were of interest largely to certain specialized groups, such as life insurance companies, for the better part of the first half of the twentieth century. A handful of studies have followed the prevalence of obesity in the United States over an extended period of time, although most data are available from about 1960 onward. In one of the few long-term studies, economist John Komlos and statistician Marek Brabec found that the BMI of selected groups of 18-year-old military cadets rose from about 19.9 during 1850–1879 to 22.3 during 1920–1939, after which it remained relatively constant until the 1980s. At that point, it began to increase dramatically to about 24.2 (Komlos and Brabec 2010). From the 1960s on, however, much more detailed and complete data are available about the prevalence of obesity in the United States.

Precisely when obesity became an issue of major importance in the United States is difficult to say. What is clear is that over the past 50 years, the rates of overweight, obesity, and morbid obesity have continued to rise at a steady pace. As Table 1.1 shows, the percentage of Americans aged 20 and above who can be defined as obese increased from 13.3 percent during 1960–1962 to 34.7 percent during 2011–2014. During the same period, the percentage of children aged 6–11 who are obese increased from 4.2 to 17.5 percent and among adolescents from 4.6 to 20.5 percent. There seems little doubt that the problem of overweight and obesity has increased substantially over the past half century in America.

In concluding the section on obesity, it should be noted that views about obesity have traditionally been held in many parts of the world other than Western Europe. Among certain tribes in Africa, for example, there is a long tradition of males' preferring obese women for their wives. In those cultures, heavy women are perceived as "the epitome of beauty and symbol of desire, prosperity, wealth, homeliness, motherliness and virtue." Obesity may also be perceived as a predictor of fertility and easy pregnancy. In order to achieve this goal, the tradition in these tribes has often been to send prospective brides

Table 1.1   Rate of Obesity, Overweight, and Healthy Weight among Americans, Aged Six and Above, 1960–2014*

Adults Aged 20 and Above

Healthy Weight

Group	1960–1962	1971–1974	1976–1980	1988–1994	1999–2002	2005–2008	2011–2014
All	51.2	48.8	49.6	41.7	32.9	30.6	28.9
Male	48.3	43.0	45.4	37.9	30.2	26.0	26.0
Female	54.1	54.3	53.7	45.3	35.6	35.1	31.7

Overweight (includes obese)

All	44.8	47.7	47.4	56.0	65.2	67.7	69.5
Male	49.5	54.7	52.9	61.0	68.8	73.0	73.0
Female	40.2	41.1	42.0	51.2	61.7	62.6	66.2

Obese

All	13.3	14.6	15.1	23.3	31.1	34.7	36.4
Male	10.7	12.2	12.8	20.6	28.1	33.3	34.5
Female	15.7	16.8	17.1	26.0	34.0	36.2	38.1

Children Aged 6–11

Obese

All	4.2	4,0	11.3	15.9	17.0	18.8	17.5
Male	4.0	4.3	11.6	16.9	18.0	20.7	17.6
Female	4.5	3.6	11.0	14.7	15.8	16.9	17.5

Adolescents Aged 12–19

Obese

All	4.6	6.1	10.5	16.0	17.6	18.2	20.5
Male	4.5	6.1	11.3	16.7	18.2	19.4	20.1
Female	4.7	6.2	9.7	15.3	16.8	16.9	21.0

Source: "Health, United States 2010." 2011. National Center for Health Statistics. https://www.cdc.gov/nchs/data/hus/hus10.pdf. Accessed on April 22, 2017; and "Health, United States 2015." 2016. National Center for Health Statistics. https://www.cdc.gov/nchs/data/hus/hus15.pdf. Accessed on April 22, 2017.

*Some definitions and year periods differ between 2010 and 2015 reports.

to a separate area known as the *fattening* (or *fatting*) *room*, where they are fed rich diets and "plumped up" for their future husbands. This cultural norm has survived to the present day among some tribes, who continue to maintain fattening rooms for their young women (The Fattening Rooms of the Efik—Culture—Nairaland 2015).

Anorexia Nervosa

Numerous accounts about anorexia nervosa (even when not mentioned by this modern term) are also available from the ancient world. The Greek historian Herodotus, for example, writes about his travels to Egypt sometime in the mid- to late fifth century BCE. He tells of an Egyptian practice of refraining from eating for a period of three days every month. That practice was based on the belief that all human disease and disorders derive from the consumption of food. As an attempt to guarantee or restore one to good health, then, it was necessary to empty the body of foods that had been eaten by the use of emetics and/or enemas (Herodotus n.d.).

There is little evidence that such practices were part of other early European cultures, such as those in ancient Greece (Bemporad 1997, 403–404). The situation in ancient Eastern culture, however, was very different. For example, the Jainist philosophy of the period, popular on the Indian subcontinent, taught that the physical body and eternal soul were entirely different from each other, with the former serving as a "prison" for the latter. One objective of Jainist religious practices, then, was for humans to find ways of helping the soul to escape from the body; the practice of self-starvation was such a mechanism. Indeed, one of the most famous early teachers of Jainism, Vardhamana Mahavira (ca. 540–470 BCE), toward the end of his life, decided to gradually reduce his intake of food to achieve the release of his soul. His program was so successful that he eventually died of starvation (Violatti 2013).

The theme of self-starvation is also found in a classic Jainist myth in which the goddess Uma (also known as Parvati or Durga) seeks to seduce the god Shiva in order to bear him a boy child. The problem is that Shiva is deeply engaged in meditation and is not interested in Uma's advances. As a last resort, Uma begins a fast that lasts 36,000 years in order to earn

Shiva's attention. At that point, she is successful, the two are married, and they do produce a young male child (Bemporad 1996). (Interestingly enough, this story is memorialized in a modern-day practice among some Indian women who undertake a fast in order to ensure that they will find a husband with whom they can have a perfect marriage, Shiva: Matchmaker God 2017.)

A similar story is told about the Indian mystic, Siddhartha Gautama, who was later to become the Buddha and the founder of Buddhism. At one point in his search for enlightenment, Gautama decided to drastically reduce his intake of food. He began to survive on the least amount of food possible and reached a point at which, according to one commentator, "he could touch his spine through his abdomen" (Bemporad 1996). After six years, however, the Buddha decided that self-starvation was not really the path to enlightenment, and he started eating normally again (The History, Philosophy and Practice of Buddhism 2016).

The notion that fasting was a path to self-understanding and enlightenment eventually made its way to the Western world, where it became a part of the religious belief known as Gnosticism. This sect drew, in part, on the traditions of the East and also on the teachings of Jesus about the practice of fasting. One of the better-known passages of the Bible tells of the temptation of Jesus by Satan in the wilderness. In that story, Jesus is said to have fasted for "forty days and forty nights," refusing every offer by Satan to break his fast by turning a stone into a loaf of bread. In the end, Jesus makes the now-famous observation: "Man shall not live on bread alone, but on every word that comes from the mouth of God" (Matthew 4:1–11; Mark 1:12–13; Luke 4:1–4).

For certain early Christian sects, then, fasting became a regular and essential aspect of their lives. As one student of the period has written, fasting was deemed appropriate for a host of occasions, including "to prepare for baptism, to mourn and commemorate Jesus' death (for many their only routine practice of fasting as a ritual act of lamentation), to better resist temptation, to obtain revelation, as part of their observance of stations, in response to persecution, and to care for the poor and address community needs and support community goals" (Rufe 1994). It apparently was not totally uncommon for early converts to Christianity to take the suggestions for self-starvation to their logical conclusion: their own deaths. According to some authorities, in fact, the first reliable report of death from the practice occurred in 383 CE, when a woman follower of Saint Jerome adopted the practice and eventually starved herself to death (Pearce 2004, 191).

Nor was fasting a minor feature of early Christian philosophy and practice. In fact, many saints of the church wrote fervently about the practice, such as the following:

- Saint Gregory: It is impossible to engage in spiritual conflict, without the previous subjugation of the appetite.
- Saint John Chrysostom: Fasting is the support of our soul . . . God, like an indulgent father, offers us a cure by fasting.
- Saint Basil: Fasting was ordained in Paradise.
- Saint Alphonsus De Ligouri: To abandon, for God's sake, all worldly enjoyments, has always been the practice of holy souls.
- Saint Leo: Fasting is always profitable both to the soul and body. (Bianchini 2014; for a list of other saints who spoke and wrote about fasting, see Secrets of the Saints: The Forgotten Spiritual Power of Fasting 2018)

Some scholars have pointed out the growing enthusiasm about fasting among Roman Catholics during the Middle Ages (or from about 1200 to about 1500). The one person who perhaps personifies this philosophy best was Caterina di Giacomo di Benincasa, later to become Saint Catherine. Born in 1347, Catherine decided at the early age of seven to "deprive herself of this flesh, of all flesh as far as possible." When her mother insisted that she join the family for meals, Catherine is said to have thrown her food under the table in order to abide by her belief about fasting (Reda and Sacco 2001). Throughout her life, Catherine continued to fast to the greatest degree possible, a practice that eventually led to her death at the age of 33. (One historian has concluded that about half of the 170 Catholic saints whom he has studied clearly demonstrated signs of anorexia. See Bell 1987.)

Catherine was by no means the only person to commit herself (rarely, himself) to self-starvation. Indeed, records now confirm the existence of substantial numbers of women who accepted self-starvation as the highest honor that they could give to Jesus and God. These women became known as the "miracle maidens," at least partly because they appeared to exist on little or no food and water for very long periods at a time. Indeed, stories of individual maidens who practice self-starvation (or, as it was called then, *anorexia mirabilis* ["miraculous lack of appetite"]) and lists of such individuals are now available in the literature. (See, e.g., Brumberg 2000, chapter 2: "From Sainthood to Patienthood"; Gutierrez 2016, chapter 5: "The Maiden Neither Eate nor Drank One Morsel or Droppe: Miracle Maidens as Colonial Objects," and Appendix III: Chronological Listing of Descriptions of Miracle Maidens Published in England, 1589–1677.) (The condition described here has also been called *holy anorexia* because women afflicted with the condition were supposedly to eat only a communion wafer, if anything at all, Bell 1987.)

By the end of the sixteenth century, views about miracle maidens and holy anorexia had become quite mixed. Many church leaders and laypersons revered these women as holy and blessed, if not actually saints, like Catherine. They visited such individuals to revere them and to ask for their blessings. But another view also became popular. As the Roman Catholic Church edged toward the Inquisition after about 1500, some church authorities saw miracle maidens not as devoted followers of Christ but as witches who used spells and rituals to achieve their remarkable lifestyles. Thus, it happened that many of the miracle maidens were eventually judged to be heretics and were burned at the stake in public ceremonies (Brumberg 2000, chapter 3).

The teachings of the saints, such as those noted earlier, have been greatly modified over the centuries but remain, in effect, in a greatly reduced form for most Roman Catholics today. The controlling ruling on this matter in the United States is provided in a Pastoral Statement on Penance and Abstinence issued by the National Conference of Catholic Bishops on November 18, 1966. According to that pronouncement, all Catholics between the ages of 18 and 59 are obligated to fast on Ash Wednesday and Good Friday (except for certain exceptions) and to be abstinent (avoiding certain specific foods, such as meats) on Fridays during Lent (Fast and Abstinence 1966).

As the period known as the Middle Ages grew to a close, the issue of self-starvation began to take on a new interpretation. With the rise of modern science in the late sixteenth and early seventeenth centuries, some observers began to view the condition less commonly as a spiritual event but in scientific terms attempting to explain the phenomenon in terms of observable and measurable physical and biological traits. Credit for the first scientific description of the condition is usually given to English physician Richard Morton. In 1694, he published the report of his examination of two adolescents, one boy and one girl, who presented with a condition he had not previously seen, a condition he referred to as *nervous consumption*. He described the signs of the condition as follows:

> A nervous atrophy or consumption, is a wasting of the body without any remarkable fever, cough, or shortness of breath; but is attended by a want of appetite, and a bad digestion, upon which there follows a languishing weakness of nature, and a falling away of the flesh every day more and more. (Morton 1694, 4)

In addition to Morton's studies, a number of physicians in the eighteenth century commented on medical conditions that appear to be those of anorexia. In the early 1700s, for example, Giorgio Baglivi, who at the time held the chair in medical theory at the Collegio della Sapienza in Rome, described a number of cases of anorexia-like conditions, for which he could find no physical cause nor cure. Interestingly enough, he hypothesized that the condition was class related. It seemed to be most common among members of the upper class who had "other things to think about than overcharging their Stomach with Gluttony and Drunkedness." Among these individuals, Baglivi wrote, "a great Part of Diseases either take their Rise from, or are fed by that Weight of Care that hangs upon every one's Shoulders." By contrast, he said, members of the lower classes were "less sensitive and better able to cope with grief and worry" (Bell 1987, 4). A similar case study was reported by English physician Robert Whytt in 1764. He described a "lad of 14 years," who, although he had no other signs or symptoms, "was observed to be low-spirited and thoughtful, to lose his appetite, and have a bad digestion." He too was unable to find a physical cause for the boy's problem and could only conclude that it was "a good instance of a nervous atrophy" (Whytt 1765, 295–296).

An important turning point in the history of eating disorders occurred in 1868, when Sir William Whitney Gull, then physician to Queen Victoria, offered a paper to the British Medical Association, meeting in Oxford, in which he provided for the first time a clear, modern definition of anorexia nervosa. In addition to his description of women he had treated for the condition, he provided a number of sketches showing patients before and after treatment, sketches that dramatically illustrated his success in dealing with the condition. Gull's contribution is important because, for the first time in history, anorexia had been distinguished from the far more commonly used term of *hysteria* to describe the symptoms of anorexia.

That term had had a long and much less-than salubrious use within the medical community dating back to ancient times. It was a kind of catch-all phrase that was used with women who did not behave according to existing social standards of the time, for which the intended cures included a wide variety of approaches, ranging from the use of herbs to forced sexual experiences. Thus, Gull's work removed the appearance of anorexia from the supernatural to the scientific, defining it, for the first time, as a psychological disorder (Gull 1997; for an excellent review of the concept of hysteria, see Tasca et al. 2012; at almost the same time as Gull's announcement, French physician Ernest Charles Lasègue issued his own report on "hysterical anorexia," apparently identical to Gull's anorexia nervosa; see Lasègue, 1997).

One of the most interesting points about anorexia has been the discovery that the condition appears to have been very rare in the pre-twentieth century or, at the very least, not extensively studied by the scientific community. That conclusion becomes clear in a review conducted in 1983 by Regina Casper at Stanford Medical School. In an extensive review of cases that could fairly definitely be described as dealing with anorexia, Dr. Casper found only about two dozen that corresponded with modern definitions and symptomology of the condition (Casper 1983, 6, table 1). Casper goes on to note that over the next 50 years, "other reports on the phenomenon of overeating in the context of fasting or dieting could not be located." In the second period reviewed by Casper, between 1900 and 1960, there were 296 cases of anorexia reported in the scientific literature corresponding to then current (1983) definitions of anorexia (Casper 1983, 8, table 2).

For nearly a century after the work of Gull and Lasègue, a new perception of anorexia became popular: it was thought of as, most likely, an endocrine disorder. The endocrine system consists of the glands that secrete a variety of hormones, which, in turn, control many different bodily functions. The early twentieth century was, in some ways, the "golden era" of endocrine research, as new hormones were discovered at a significant rate, and the wide variety of functions carried out by these hormones was discovered (for an excellent review of this period, see Harrower 1932, 21–41).

One of the hypotheses developed during this period was that anorexia was caused by a hormone deficiency or hormone malfunction. This hypothesis grew out of the research of German pathologist Morris Simmonds in 1914 on several women who had died of cachexia. Cachexia is a wasting disorder characterized by loss of weight, muscle atrophy, fatigue, weakness, and significant loss of appetite. The condition comes about not as the result of someone's trying to lose weight but because of some bodily abnormality. Because of the involvement of the pituitary gland, the technical name for the condition is *hypopituitarism*, a less-than-normal (*hypo-*) functioning of the pituitary gland. The condition is also known by a number of other names, including Simmonds' disorder, Glinski-Simmonds syndrome, Reye-Sheehan syndrome, Simmonds-Sheehan syndrome, Simmonds cachexia, Simmonds syndrome, and Reye's syndrome.

Some medical workers soon made a connection between Simmonds' disorder and anorexia because the symptoms of the two conditions were so similar. This similarity prompted a number of physicians to begin treating women with anorexia with a variety of hormones, including insulin, thyroxine, follicle-stimulating hormone, luteinizing hormone, estrogen, and adrenocorticotropic hormone. Some of these hormones appeared to have some beneficial effects on some women, prompting the medical profession to continue this line of research (Summers 1947).

Research on and treatment for anorexia followed the endocrine line of thinking for most of the first half of the twentieth century. In the 1940s, however, some researchers began to question whether anorexia was really a hormone-based condition. In 1942, for example, John M. Berkman at the Mayo Clinic in Rochester, Minnesota, found that only about 16 percent of the patients treated by Simmonds with hormones had true pituitary lesions, thus qualifying for a diagnosis of Simmonds' disease. The remaining 84 percent died from some wasting condition other than Simmonds' disease (Berkman, Weir, and Kepler 1947). Shortly thereafter, British pathologists H. L. Sheehan and V. K. Summers reported that patients with anorexia nervosa on the one hand and Simmonds' disease on the other actually had only two characteristics in common: extreme weight loss and an intense motivation to become thin (Sheehan and Summers 1949).

Research on possible connections between hormonal dysfunction and anorexia did not come to an end with the abandonment of the Simmonds–anorexia connection in the late 1940s. Indeed, reports of such research have continued to the present day (see, e.g., Miller 2013). Over time, however, experts in the field slowly began to acknowledge the psychological and emotional factors responsible for the development of anorexia. One of the earliest and most powerful books on this topic was *Eating Disorders: Obesity, Anorexia Nervosa, and the Person Within*, by German-born American psychotherapist Hilde Bruch. Bruch opened her book by reviewing historical theories of and treatment of anorexia before acknowledging that eating disorders are not fundamentally disorders of the human body but "reciprocal transactional processes with the interpersonal field," that is, ways in which individuals react with and respond to their relationships with other (Bruch 1974, 5).

An indication of the status of anorexia (and other eating disorders) in the second half of the twentieth century can be found in various editions of the *Diagnostic and Statistical Manual of Mental Disorders* (*DSM*) of the American Psychiatric Association. The *DSM* is the standard reference source in the United States for defining the symptoms of all mental disorders recognized by the psychiatric profession. The first edition of the *DSM* (*DSM-I*) was published in 1952, and it made only passing mention of anorexia or any other eating disorder. *DSM-II* was published in 1968 and also provided only a modest view of the condition. It was listed in this edition as a "special condition" that did not fit into any other category of disorders, where it was described as a "feeding disturbance" (Committee on Nomenclature and Statistics of the American Psychiatric Association 1968, 47–48). The second edition of the *DSM* did not go much further in terms of providing information and guidance about the disorder (Dell'Osso et al. 2016).

The third edition of the *DSM* (*DSM-III*), published in 1980, finally had a more extensive section on anorexia under the category "Disorders Usually First Evident in Infancy, Childhood, or Adolescence." This classification was justified because anorexia was then thought (incorrectly) to be a disorder that could affect a person at any age but that it was much more common to first appear during childhood. The diagnostic criteria for anorexia as provided in *DSM-III* are as follows:

A. Intense fear of becoming obese, which does not diminish as weight loss progresses.

B. Disturbance of body image, e.g., claiming to "feel fat" even when emaciated.

C. Weight loss of at least 25% of original body weight or, if under 18 years of age, weight loss from original body weight plus projected weight gain expected from growth charts may be combined to make the 25%.

D. Refusal to maintain body weight over a minimal normal weight for age and height.

E. No known physical illness that would account for the weight loss. (*Diagnostic and Statistical Manual of Mental Disorders* 1980, 69)

DSM-IV published in 1994 an even more specific description of the criteria for anorexia nervosa:

a. Refusal to maintain body weight at or above a minimally normal weight for age and height (e.g. weight loss leading to maintenance of body weight less than 85% of that expected; or failure to make expected weight gain during period of growth, leading to body weight less than 85% of that expected).

b. Intense fear of gaining weight or becoming fat, even though underweight.

c. Disturbance in the way in which one's body weight or shape is experienced, undue influence of body weight or shape on self-evaluation, or denial of the seriousness of the current low body weight.

d. In postmenarcheal females, amenorrhoea, i.e. the absence of at least three consecutive menstrual cycles. (A woman is considered to have amenorrhoea if her periods occur only following hormone, e.g. oestrogen, administration.) (Appendix 17: Diagnostic Criteria for Eating Disorders 2004)

The most recent edition of the *DSM* has yet another version of the criteria for anorexia nervosa, the version that is currently used by experts in the field in diagnosing the condition:

A. Restriction of energy intake relative to requirements, leading to a significantly low body weight in the context of age, sex, developmental trajectory, and physical health. Significantly low weight is defined as a weight that is less than minimally normal or, for children and adolescents, less than that minimally expected.

B. Intense fear of gaining weight or of becoming fat, or persistent behavior that interferes with weight gain, even though at a significantly low weight.

C. Disturbance in the way in which one's body weight or shape is experienced, undue influence of body weight or shape on self-evaluation, or persistent lack of recognition of the seriousness of the current low body weight. (*Diagnostic Criteria for Eating Disorders— DSM V* 2015)

Bulimia Nervosa

Bulimia was first identified as a unique and definable mental disorder by British psychiatrist Gerald Russell in 1979. In his now-famous paper on the topic, "Bulimia Nervosa: An Ominous Variant of Anorexia Nervosa," Russell argued that at least two different forms of anorexia existed, one in which the primary mechanism was self-starvation (anorexia) and the other binging and purging. He said that the two conditions were sufficiently different from each other to deserve different psychological, medical, and psychiatric categorization. He then proposed the term *bulimia nervosa* (originally meaning "ox [*bous*] hunger [*limous*]" or, somewhat later "ravenous hunger," in Greek). In his paper, Russell looked back over the long history of eating disorders and selected specific examples of cases in which a person could better be diagnosed as *bulimic* than as *anorexic* (Giles 2012).

The practice of intentionally vomiting after eating among the ancient Egyptians, in order to maintain one's health (noted earlier), for example, is probably better described as a type of bulimic reaction than anorexia. Historians have chosen a number of reports of bulimic-like behaviors in history also. Galen, for example, described a condition that he named *bulimis* in which an individual ate to excess and then relieved himself or herself by vomiting (Cassell and Gleaves 2006, xvii). In suggesting that bulimia may be both a historical and intercultural phenomenon, two scholars at the University of California, Irvine, reported in 1994 that they believed that bulimia may have been an inherent part of the culture of residents of the Trobriand Islands, in the Pacific Ocean. They report that one member of the society had been quoted as saying that "we shall be glad [when the spare season had passed], we shall eat until we vomit" (although it is not clear from this article that the practice actually met the modern criteria for a bulimic experience; see Blinder and Chao 1994). The scholars then went on to review a number of other cases of bulimia that were reported in the scientific literature from 1800 through 1994. One interesting comment about the research is that the distinction between anorexia and bulimia was not at all clear throughout that period. They cite one study that suggests that 43 percent of the cases of anorexia that had been reviewed actually met the modern criteria for bulimia also, thus making it essentially impossible to know how those cases would be categorized today (Casper et al. 1980, 1034).

The modern history of bulimia can probably be traced to the 1940s, when reports of the condition mention symptoms that are now well known to be characteristic of the condition. Probably the most famous of those cases was described by Swiss psychiatrist Ludwig Binswanger in 1944. The case involved a young woman, Ellen West, who was obsessed from early in her life by fears of gaining weight. Eventually, these fears became more generalized and so unbearable that she committed suicide in 1921 at the age of 33. Her story is of particular interest because she kept a very detailed diary of her thoughts, feelings, and experiences while trying to work her way thought her obsessions about food (Furst 2015).

Perhaps the most interesting question of all with regard to bulimia is how common the condition has been throughout history. Certainly, very few scientific studies of the condition appeared prior to 1960, although the number of cases reported after that date has increased quite steadily and sometimes quite dramatically. These observations have led one observer in the field to ask "whether or not bulimia was observed and had existed as a clinical entity before 1960, and what kind of factors could have contributed to its recent rise" (Casper 1983, 4).

Certainly, the psychiatric profession had little to say about the condition prior to the release of the third edition of the *Diagnostic and Statistical Manual of Mental Disorders* in 1980. Neither *DSM-I* nor *DSM-II* had any mention of the disorder, although it was finally mention and defined, along with characteristic symptoms, in *DSM-III*. According to that document, the diagnostic criteria for bulimia are as follows:

A. Recurrent episodes of binge eating (rapid consumption of a large amount of food in a discrete period of time, usually less than two hours).

B. At least three of the following:

1. consumption of high-caloric, easily ingested food during a binge

2. inconspicuous eating during a binge

3. termination of such eating episodes by abdominal pain, sleep, social interruption, or self-induced vomiting

4. repeated attempts to lose weight by severely restrictive diets, self-induced vomiting, or use of cathartics or diuretics

5. frequent weight fluctuations greater than ten pounds due to alternating binges and fasts

C. Awareness that the eating pattern is abnormal and fear of not being able to stop eating voluntarily.

D. Depressed mood and self-deprecating thoughts following eating binges.

E. The bulimic episodes are not due to Anorexia Nervosa or any known physical disorder. (*Diagnostic and Statistical Manual of Mental Disorders* 1980, 70–71)

The formal definition for bulimia today is now contained in the latest edition of the manual, *DSM-V*, released in 2013, which says that bulimia can be recognized by the following:

A. Recurrent episodes of binge eating. An episode of binge eating is characterized by both of the following:

1. Eating, in a discrete period of time (e.g., within any two-hour period), an amount of food that is definitely larger than most people would eat

during a similar period of time and under similar circumstances.

2. A sense of lack of control over eating during the episode (e.g., a feeling that one cannot stop eating or control what or how much one is eating).

B. Recurrent inappropriate compensatory behavior to prevent weight gain, such as self-induced vomiting; misuse of laxatives, diuretics, enemas, or other medications; fasting; or excessive exercise.

C. The binge eating and inappropriate compensatory behaviors both occur, on average, at least once a week for three months.

D. Self-evaluation is unduly influenced by body shape and weight.

E. The disturbance does not occur exclusively during episodes of anorexia nervosa. (*Diagnostic Criteria for Eating Disorders—DSM V* 2015)

Other Eating Disorders

There is a fairly dramatic change in the discussion of eating disorders between the release of *DSM-IV* in 1994 and *DSM-V*, nearly two decades later, in 2013. The treatment of eating disorders was significantly expanded, and some new categories were introduced. The types of eating disorders now listed in *DSM-V* are the following:

• Anorexia nervosa
• Bulimia nervosa
• Binge eating disorder
• Pica
• Rumination disorder
• Avoidant/restrictive food intake disorder
• Other specified feeding or eating disorder
• Unspecified feeding or eating disorder

(Other types of eating disorders not formally recognized by medical groups also exist. They include bigorexia, body dysmorphic disorder, night-eating syndrome, orthorexia, pica, Prader-Willi syndrome, and sleeping-eating disorder. See, e.g., Other Types of Eating Disorders 2016.)

A brief explanation of each *DSM* category is as follows:

Binge Eating Disorder

A type of eating disorder only recently identified is BED. The condition was first described in a now-famous paper by psychiatrist Albert J. Strunk of the Hospital of the University of Pennsylvania in 1959. Strunk drew on research of mice, who were provided with varying types of feeding plants. He noted that in some cases, mice would binge by eating very large amounts of food in a short time on an irregular basis throughout an experiment. The consequence of this feeding pattern was that mice became obese and developed a number of weight-related illnesses. Strunk hypothesized that the same type of eating patterns might also occur in humans. He identified three characteristics of the pattern observed among humans: (1) a pattern of "night-eating" that was followed by anorexia the next day, insomnia, hyperphagia (an abnormal increase in appetite); (2) binge eating that occurs at irregular intervals; and (3) failure to reach satiation, that is, continuing to feel hungry even after eating large amounts of food. Stunkard himself used the term *night-eating syndrome* (*NES*) for this phenomenon (Stunkard 1959).

Over the next three decades, NES was studied in more detail, and a clearer understanding of the precise character of the disorder developed among psychiatrists. The profession first formally recognized the behavior in *DSM-III*, when it was listed as part of the description of bulimia nervosa. In the next edition of the manual, *DSM-IV*, BED was moved to a new category, "eating disorder not otherwise specified" (EDNOS), a catch-all category that included any type of eating disorder that did not fit under anorexia or bulimia. Finally, BED received its own section in *DSM-V* with a set of symptoms by which it can be recognized:

- Eating much more rapidly than normal
- Eating until feeling uncomfortably full
- Eating large amounts of food when not feeling physically hungry
- Eating alone because of being embarrassed by how much one is eating
- Feeling disgusted with oneself, depressed, or very guilty after overeating (Berkman et al. 2015, table 1).

Pica

Pica is an eating disorder characterized by the desire, even preference, for substances that are not usually thought as foods, such as ashes, chalk, cigarette ashes, clay and other forms of dirt, coffee grounds, hair, paint chips, plaster, soap, and other materials that cannot be digested and have no nutritional value. It is a condition that occurs most commonly among infants, children, and individuals with developmental disabilities (Barkoukis, Reiss, and Dombeck 2008). As with so many other medical conditions, the first mention of pica appears to occur in the writings of the Roman physician Galen. In his work *Practical Physik*, he writes of women of about 50 years of age who "desire strange and absurd things," such as coal and ashes. He also associates pica with another common illness, *greensickness*, known among such women (Sennertus, Culpeper, and Cole 1664, 46, 71, 101, 163). The term *pica* comes from the Latin word *pīca*, meaning "magpie." The choice of names apparently reflects that bird's tendency to be attracted to and carry away a wide variety of materials and objects in its nest-building activities (T. E. C., Jr., 1969, 548).

Galen also associated pica with a condition known as greensickness, which he describes as "the changing of the natural colour into a pale and green with Faintness, Heaviness of Body,

Loathing of Meat, Palpitation of the Heart, difficult Breathing, Sadness, Swelling of the Feet, Eyelids, and Face, from depraved Nourishment" (Sennertus, Culpeper, and Cole 1664, 100; Galen devotes all of chapter 2 to a discussion of this condition; he also refers to the disorder as *virgins disease* and the *white fever*).

Greensickness and pica were apparently quite common among young, unmarried women of the seventeenth century. Historians have often related these conditions to the modern phenomenon of love sickness. The condition was most commonly associated with a woman's virginity or menstrual state and was serious enough to lead to madness. One specific example of this state was *Hamlet*'s Ophelia, who has thought to have displayed the symptoms of greensickness and eventually gone made as a consequence of the disorder (Dawson 2008, chapter 2). A later, more complete, medical definition is attributed to French surgeon Ambrose Paré in 1588.

For most of the period from 1600 to the late twentieth century, medical specialists thought of pica as a symptom of other mental and emotional disorders but not as a unique condition in and of itself (for an excellent review of this period, see Mayes 1992, chapter 7). That policy changed in 1994 when pica was provided with its own discrete categorization code 307.52, which described the condition as one characterized by the following:

A. Persistent eating of nonnutritive substances for a period of at least 1 month.

B. The eating of nonnutritive substances is inappropriate to the developmental level.

C. The eating behavior is not part of a culturally sanctioned practice.

D. If the eating behavior occurs exclusively during the course of another mental disorder (e.g., Mental Retardation, Pervasive Developmental Disorder, Schizophrenia), it is sufficiently severe to warrant independent clinical attention. (Diagnostic Criteria for 307.52 Pica 2017; this definition was changed in *DSM-IV*)

Rumination Disorder

The most common context in which the word *rumination* is encountered is probably in a discussion of certain mammals that regurgitate the food they have eaten, chew that food a second time, and then continue digesting the food. Among the more than 150 animals that ruminate their food are antelopes, camels, cows, bison, deer, giraffes, moose, sheep, water buffalo, and yaks. Rumination in humans also occurs, most commonly among children. The phenomenon was first described in 1618 by Italian anatomist Fabricius ab Aquapendente, who wrote of encountering the phenomenon in two of his patients. Interestingly enough, Fabricius noted that one of his two ruminant patients had two horns growing out of his forehead, while the other was the son of a man who had had one horn. (Of the many historical mentions of this phenomenon, see Copland 1821.) Rumination was also once known as *merycism*, from the Greek word for *rumination*. (For more on the early history of rumination, see Brockbank 1907.)

The mention of a horn or horns in association with the phenomenon of rumination continued through much of the literature up to the proper time. The occurrence of such horns appears to be possible and have been called *cutaneous horns* by the medical profession (Human Horns: A Dilemma for Some, A Delight for Others 2017; Tubbs et al. 2003). There is no evidence, however, that such anatomical features have any relationship whatsoever with the phenomenon of rumination disorders. Although anatomical features were apparently of considerable interest to the medical profession when cases of rumination were observed, the actual frequency of the phenomenon appears to have been low. In a survey of the mention of human rumination in an 1894 review article, for example, the author claims to have found fewer than 50 well-documented cases in all of medical history to that date (Einhorn 1890; Sinkler 1898).

The medical community seems never to have quite known how to treat rumination. It was often considered simply to be an oddity of human behavior, and people who engaged in the activity were sometimes exhibited at circuses. During the early twentieth century, studies of rumination usually focused on its appearance among infants, children, and the mentally retarded. Only after the middle of the century did scholars begin thinking of the disorder in terms of a psychological issue found in specific, often adult, individuals (Parry-Jones 1994). Finally, in *DSM-III*, rumination was listed as a disorder first evident in infants, children, or adolescents. It was described as a condition in which someone in this age group regurgitated food and then swallowed the food once more, without obvious nausea (*Diagnostic and Statistical Manual of Mental Disorders* 1980, 72–73). The description of rumination was then revised for both *DSM-IV* and *DSM-V*, in the latter case to make it clear that the condition could at any time in an individual's life (Black and Grant 2014, 220).

Avoidant/Restrictive Food Intake Disorder

Avoidant/restrictive food intake disorder is among the newest of all eating disorders. The term was first used in *DSM-V* in place of a *DSM-IV* category known as *feeding disorder of infancy or early childhood*. One of the major reasons for the new term was that the condition it describes was rarely used by professionals in the field, and little study had been on ARFID. Because of this fact, very little was known about the individuals who were diagnosed with or thought to have this type of eating disorder (*Diagnostic and Statistical Manual of Mental Disorders: DSM-5* 2013, 35–37). The category includes a number of eating behaviors that are not clearly identifiable as anorexia, bulimia, pica, or another named disorder. The subcategories of ARFID are atypical anorexia nervosa, BED, bulimia nervosa of low frequency and/or limited duration, purging disorder, and night-eating syndrome. Symptoms of ARFID include the rejection of food primarily because of its physical qualities (e.g., texture or taste) that results in a significant weight loss, often resulting in nutrient-inadequate diets. The new name for the condition also acknowledges that fact that a pattern of food rejection described by the *DSM-V* criteria occurs in individuals of all ages, not just children and adolescents. The condition can be serious and even life threatening because of the patient's failure to ingest a necessary range of nutrients and experience serious weight loss (Krepie and Palomaki 2012; Norris et al. 2014).

Other Specified Feeding and Eating Disorders

Like ARFID, the category of OSFED first appeared in *DSM-V*. It replaced a category in *DSM-IV* called EDNOS. OSFED is something of a "catch-all" category that includes eating disorders that may resemble anorexia, bulimia, or other disorders but does not meet all the criteria for these categories. A psychiatrist may place a patient into this category with a further indication of the way in which that person's eating disorder is similar to another category, such as atypical anorexia nervosa or low-level bulimia nervosa. Authorities in the field now believe that EDNOS is the most common of all forms of eating disorder in the United States. Studies have shown that the rate of EDNOS in the United States is 2 to 30 times that for anorexia and 2 to 3 times that of bulimia (Fairburn and Bohn 2005; Thomas, Vartanian, and Brownell 2009).

Conclusion

Eating disorders have been observed among humans almost from the moment civilized societies first appeared. Some of the descriptions provided by ancient writers are similar to those used for cases observed today. However, psychiatrists and other professionals have gradually developed more specific definitions for about a half dozen forms of eating disorders. These definitions aid specialists in recognizing the precise nature of an eating disorder, some possible causes for its appearances, and methods that can be used for its treatment.

References

"Appendix 17: Diagnostic Criteria for Eating Disorders." 2004. National Center for Biotechnology Information. https://www.ncbi.nlm.nih.gov/books/NBK49317/. Accessed on April 24, 2017.

Ashley, Wendy. 2007. "Obesity in the Body of Christ." SBC Life. http://www.sbclife.net/Articles/2007/01/sla8. Accessed on April 17, 2017.

Atwater, W. O., C. D. Woods, and F. G. Benedict. 1897. "Report of Preliminary Investigations on the Metabolism of Nitrogen and Carbon in the Human Organism." U.S. Department of Agriculture. http://ufdc.ufl.edu/AA0001 4628/00001/1j. Accessed on April 21, 2017.

Banting, William. 1864. *Letter on Corpulence*. London: Harrison.

Barkoukis, Andrea, Natalie Staats Reiss, and Mark Dombeck. 2008. "Feeding and Eating Disorders of Infancy or Early Childhood: Pica." MentalHealth.net. https://www.mentalhelp.net/articles/feeding-and-eating-disorders-of-infancy-or-early-childhood-pica/. Accessed on May 22, 2017.

Bell, Rudolph M. 1987. *Holy Anorexia*. Chicago, IL: University of Chicago Press.

Bemporad, Jules R. 1996. "Self-Starvation through the Ages: Reflections on the Pre-history of Anorexia Nervosa." *International Journal of Eating Disorders*. 19(3): 217–237. http://docshare02.docshare.tips/files/29910/299108865.pdf. Accessed on April 10, 2017.

Bemporad, Jules R. 1997. "Cultural and Historical Aspects of Eating Disorders." *Theoretical Medicine*. 18(4): 401–420. http://brown.uk.com/eatingdisorders/bemporad.pdf. Accessed on April 10, 2017.

Berkman, J. M., J. F. Weir, and E. J. Kepler. 1947. "Clinical Observations on Starvation Edema, Serum Protein and the Effect of Forced Feeding in Anorexia Nervosa." *Gastroenterology*. 9(4): 357–390.

Berkman, N. D., et al. 2015. "Comparative Effectiveness Reviews, No. 160." *Management and Outcomes of Binge-Eating Disorder*. Rockville, MD: Agency for Healthcare Research and Quality. https://www.ncbi.nlm.nih.gov/books/NBK338301/table/introduction.t1/. Accessed on April 26, 2017.

Berryman, Jack W. 2012. "Motion and Rest: Galen on Exercise and Health." *The Lancet*. 380(9838): 210–211.

Bianchini, Davide A. 2014. "The Case for the Restoration of Fasting in Religious Life." Religious Vocation. http://www.religious-vocation.com/fasting_religious_renewal.html#.WOwCamnyupo. Accessed on April 10, 2017.

Bivins, Roberta, and Hilary Marland. 2016. "Weighting for Health: Management, Measurement and Self-Surveillance in the Modern Household." *Social History of Medicine*. 29(4): 757–780. https://academic.oup.com/shm/article/29/4/757/2660184/Weighting-for-Health-Management-Measurement-and. Accessed on April 21, 2017.

Black, Donald W., and Jon E. Grant. 2014. *DSM-5 Guidebook: The Essential Companion to the Diagnostic and Statistical Manual of Mental Disorders, Fifth Edition*. Washington, DC: American Psychiatric Publishing.

Blinder, Barton J., and Karin H. Chao. 1994. "Bulimia Nervosa/Obesity: A Historical Overview." http://www.ltspeed.com/bjblinder/publications/bulimiahistory.htm. Accessed on April 25, 2017.

"Body Mass Index." 2015. Centers for Disease Control and Prevention. https://www.cdc.gov/healthyweight/assessing/bmi/. Accessed on April 19, 2017.

Bray, George A. 1993a. "Commentary on Atwater Classic." *Obesity Research*. 1(3): 223–227. http://onlinelibrary .wiley.com/doi/10.1002/j.1550-8528.1993.tb00615.x/pdf. Accessed on April 21, 2017.

Bray, George A. 1993b. "Commentary on Classics in Obesity 5. Fat Cell Theory and Units of Knowledge." *Obesity Research*. 1(5): 403–407.

Bray, George A., and Claude Bouchard, eds. 2014. *Handbook of Obesity*, 4th ed. 2 vols. Boca Raton, FL: CRC Press.

Brockbank, E. M. 1907. "Merycism or Rumination in Man." *British Medical Journal*. 1(2408): 421–427.

Bruch, Hilde. 1974. *Eating Disorders: Obesity, Anorexia Nervosa, and the Person Within*. London: Routledge & Kegan Paul.

Brumberg, Joan Jacobs. 2000. *Fasting Girls: The History of Anorexia Nervosa*. New York: Random House; London: Hi Marketing.

Casper, Regina C. 1983. "On the Emergence of Bulimia Nervosa as a Syndrome: A Historical View." *International Journal of Eating Disorders*. 2(3): 3–16.

Casper, Regina C., et al. 1980. "Bulimia. Its Incidence and Clinical Importance in Patients with Anorexia Nervosa." *Archives of General Psychiatry*. 37(9): 1030–1035.

Cassell, Dana K., and David H. Gleaves. 2006. *The Encyclopedia of Obesity and Eating Disorders*. New York: Facts on File.

Cheyne, George. 1724. "An Essay of Health and Long Life." Eighteenth Century Collection Online. http://quod.lib .umich.edu/e/ecco/004834818.0001.000?rgn=main;view= fulltext. Accessed on April 17, 2017.

Christopoulou-Aletra, Helen, and Niki Papavramidou. 2004. "Methods Used by the Hippocratic Physicians for Weight Reduction." *World Journal of Surgery.* 28(5): 513–517. https://www.academia.edu/4815859/Methods_Used_ by_the_Hippocratic_Physicians_for_Weight_Reduction. Accessed on April 14, 2017.

Committee on Nomenclature and Statistics of the American Psychiatric Association. 1968. *Diagnostic and Statistical Manual of Mental Disorders* ("DSM-II"). Washington, DC: American Psychiatric Association. http://www.behavior ismandmentalhealth.com/wp-content/uploads/2015/08/ DSM-II.pdf. Accessed on April 24, 2017.

Copland, James. 1821. "History of a Case of Human Rumination." *The London Medical and Physical Journal.* 45: 362–374. https://books.google.com/books?id=Ej0CAAAA YAAJ&pg=PA371&lpg=PA371&dq=rumination+fabricus& source=bl&ots=Z0ATU4tWEq&sig=LAOGSyJhm4cVdP TAqnsJJl2qv2U&hl=en&sa=X&ved=0ahUKEwiQn9O1k cjTAhXmllQKHXeCA2YQ6AEILTAB#v=onepage&q=ru mination%20fabricus&f=false. Accessed on April 28, 2017.

Daley, Bill. 2015. "Brillat-Savarin's Gastronomic Gem Resonates Nearly 200 Years Later." *Chicago Tribune.* http:// www.chicagotribune.com/dining/recipes/sc-food-0116- giants-brillat-savarin-20150113-story.html. Accessed on April 20, 2017.

Dawson, Lesel. 2008. *Lovesickness and Gender in Early Modern English Literature.* Oxford, UK: Oxford University Press.

Dell'Osso, Liliana, et al. 2016. "Historical Evolution of the Concept of Anorexia Nervosa and Relationships with Orthorexia Nervosa, Autism, and Obsessive—Compulsive Spectrum." *Neuropsychiatric Disease and Treatment.* 12: 1651–1660. https://www.ncbi.nlm.nih.gov/pmc/articles/ PMC4939998/. Accessed on April 24, 2017.

Diagnostic and Statistical Manual of Mental Disorders
("DSM-III"). 1980. Washington, DC: American
Psychiatric Association. http://displus.sk/DSM/subory/
dsm3.pdf. Accessed on April 24, 2017.

Diagnostic and Statistical Manual of Mental Disorders: DSM-5.
2013. Washington, DC; London: American Psychiatric
Publishing.

"Diagnostic Criteria for Eating Disorders—DSM V." 2015.
Pri-Med. http://www.pri-med.com/DigitalAssets/Shared%
20Files/Spring%202015%20Syllabus%20Files/Annnual-
Southwest%202015/Eating%20Disorders%20Handout
.pdf. Accessed on April 24, 2017.

"Diagnostic Criteria for 307.52 Pica." 2017. BehaveNet.
http://behavenet.com/node/21492. Accessed on April 27,
2017.

Dixson, Alan F., and Barnaby J. Dixson. 2011. "Venus
Figurines of the European Paleolithic: Symbols of Fertility
or Attractiveness?" *Journal of Anthropology.* 2011: 11 pages.
http://dx.doi.org/10.1155/2011/569120. https://www
.hindawi.com/journals/janthro/2011/569120/cta/.
Accessed on April 9, 2017.

Eades, Michael. 2007. "Obesity in Egypt." The Blog of
Michael R. Eades, M.D. https://proteinpower.com/drmike/
2007/07/01/obesity-in-ancient-egypt/. Accessed on April 13,
2017.

Edwardes, Charlotte. 2003. "Mr. Banting's Old Diet
Revolution." *Telegraph.* http://www.telegraph.co.uk/news/
uknews/1441407/Mr-Bantings-Old-Diet-Revolution.html.
Accessed on April 21, 2017.

Einhorn, Max. 1890. *Rumination in Man.* New York: Trow's
Printing and Bookbinding Co.

Eknoyan, Garabed. 2006. "A History of Obesity, or How
What Was Good Became Ugly and Then Bad." *Advances*

in Chronic Kidney Disease. 13(4): 421–427. http://www
.ackdjournal.org/article/S1548-5595(06)00106-6/pdf.
Accessed on April 16, 2017.

Eknoyan, Garabed. 2008. "Adolphe Quetelet (1796–1874)—
The Average Man and Indices of Obesity." *Nephrology
Dialysis Transplantation.* 23(1): 47–51.

Fairburn, Christopher G., and Kristin Bohn. 2005. "Eating
Disorder NOS (EDNOS): An Example of the Troublesome
'Not Otherwise Specified' (NOS) Category in DSM-IV."
Behaviour Research and Therapy. 43(6): 691–701.

Fairburn, Christopher G., and Kelly D. Brownell. 2005.
Eating Disorders and Obesity: A Comprehensive Handbook,
2nd ed. New York; London: Guilford. https://www.ncbi
.nlm.nih.gov/pmc/articles/PMC2785872/. Accessed on
April 29, 2017.

"Fast and Abstinence." 1966. United States Conference
of Catholic Bishops. http://www.usccb.org/prayer-and-
worship/liturgical-year/lent/catholic-information-on-
lenten-fast-and-abstinence.cfm. Accessed on April 11,
2017.

"The Fattening Rooms of the Efik—Culture—Nairaland."
2015. Nairaland. http://www.nairaland.com/2097222/
fattening-rooms-efik. Accessed on April 15, 2017.

Fish, Henry Clay. 1867. *The Agent's Manual of Life Assurance.*
Pittsfield, MS: Berkshire Life Insurance Co. https://archive
.org/details/agentsmanualofli00fishiala. Accessed on
April 21, 2017.

Flemyng, Malcolm. 1757. *A Discourse on the Nature, Causes,
and Cure of Corpulency.* London: L. Davis and C. Reymers.
http://quod.lib.umich.edu/e/ecco/004834495.0001.000?
rgn=main;view=fulltext. Accessed on April 19, 2017.

Furst, Lilian R. 2015. "The Elusive Patient and Her
Ventriloquist Therapist: Ludwig Binswanger's 'The Case of
Ellen West.'" In Lilian R. Furst, ed. *Just Talk: Narratives*

of Psychotherapy, chapter 13, 193–209. Lexington: The University Press of Kentucky.

Galen. 1662. "Tractatus de Tumoribus Praeter Naturam." Trans. by Robert Bayfield. University of Oxford. http:// tei.it.ox.ac.uk/tcp/Texts-HTML/free/A27/A27078.html. Accessed on April 15, 2017.

Galenus, Claudius, and Rudolph E. Siegel. 1976. *Galen on the Affected Parts: Translation from the Greek Text with Explanatory Notes*. Basel: S. Karger.

Giles, Chrissie. 2012. "A Burst from the Blue—Is Bulimia Nervosa Really a Modern Disease?" Wellcome Trust. https:// blog.wellcome.ac.uk/2012/02/20/a-burst-from-the-blue-is-bulimia-nervosa-really-a-modern-disease/. Accessed on April 26, 2017.

Groves, Barry. 2003. "William Banting Father of the Low-Carbohydrate Diet." The Weston A. Price Foundation. https://www.westonaprice.org/health-topics/know-your-fats/william-banting-father-of-the-low-carbohydrate-diet/. Accessed on April 21, 2017.

Gull, William W. 1997. "Anorexia Nervosa (Apepsia Hysterica, Anorexia Hysterica)" (reprint of his 1873 paper). *Obesity Research*. 5(5): 498–502. http://onlinelibrary.wiley .com/doi/10.1002/j.1550-8528.1997.tb00677.x/pdf. Accessed on April 12, 207.

Gutierrez, Nancy A. 2016. *"Shall She Famish Then?": Female Food Refusal in Early Modern England*. London: Routledge.

Harrower, Henry R. 1932. *Practical Endocrinology*, 2nd ed. Glendale, CA: Pioneer Printing Company. https://www .seleneriverpress.com/images/pdfs/0_PRACTICAL_ENDO CRINOLOGY_1932_HARROWER.pdf. Accessed on April 22, 2017.

Haslam, David W., and Fiona Haslam. 2009. *Fat, Gluttony, and Sloth: Obesity in Medicine, Art and Literature*. Liverpool: Liverpool University Press.

Hassall, Arthur. 1849. "Observations on the Development of the Fat Vesicle." *The Lancet*. 53(1325): 63–64.

Hassall, Arthur Hill. 1851. *The Microscopic Anatomy of the Human Body, in Health and Disease*. New York: Pratt, Woodford & Co. https://ia800309.us.archive.org/30/items/microscopicanato12hass/microscopicanato12hass.pdf. Accessed on April 20, 2017.

Herodotus. n.d. "An Account of Egypt." Project Gutenberg. https://www.gutenberg.org/files/2131/2131-h/2131-h.htm. Accessed on April 10, 2017.

Hippocrates. 1868. "Aphorisms." Trans. by Charles Darwin Adams. Digital Hippocrates. http://classics.mit.edu/Hippocrates/aphorisms.1.i.html. Accessed on November 27, 2018.

"The History, Philosophy and Practice of Buddhism." 2016. https://www.buddha101.com/h_life.htm. Accessed on April 10, 2017.

Holloway, April. 2014. "The Venus Figurines of the Paleolithic Era." Ancient Origins. http://www.ancient-origins.net/ancient-places-europe/venus-figurines-european-paleolithic-era-001548. Accessed on April 9, 2017.

"Human Horns: A Dilemma for Some, a Delight for Others." 2017. Web Ecoist. http://webecoist.momtastic.com/2010/05/11/human-horns-a-dilemma-for-some-a-delight-for-others/. Accessed on April 28, 2017.

Józsa, László G. 2011. "Obesity in the Paleolithic Era." *Hormones*. 10(3): 241–244.

Katch, Frank I. 1999. "Wilbur Olin Atwater (1844–1907)." History Makers. http://www.sportsci.org/news/history/atwater/atwater.html. Accessed on April 21, 2017.

Komaroff, Marina. 2016. "For Researchers on Obesity: Historical Review of Extra Body Weight Definitions."

Journal of Obesity. 2016: 1–9. https://www.hindawi.com/journals/jobe/2016/2460285/#B19. Accessed on April 21, 2017.

Komlos, John, and Marek Brabec. 2010. "The Evolution of BMI Values of US Adults: 1882–1986." VOX. http://voxeu.org/article/100-years-us-obesity. Accessed on April 21, 2017.

Krepie, Richard E., and Angela Palomaki. 2012. "Beyond Picky Eating: Avoidant/Restrictive Food Intake Disorder." *Current Psychiatry Reports*. 14(4): 421–431.

Lasègue, Ernest-Charles. 1997. "On Hysterical Anorexia (a)." *Obesity Research*. 5(5): 492–497. http://onlinelibrary.wiley.com/doi/10.1002/j.1550-8528.1997.tb00676.x/epdf. Accessed on April 22, 2017.

Mayes, Susan Dickerson. 1992. "Eating Disorders of Infancy and Early Childhood." In Stephen R. Hooper, George W. Hynd, and Richard E. Mattison, eds. *Child Psychopathology: Diagnostic Criteria and Clinical Assessment*, chapter 7, 203–260. Hoboken, NJ: Taylor and Francis.

Maynard, Philip. 2010. *The Jesus Diet: An Easy Way for Christians to Lose Weight*. Bloomington, IN: CrossBooks.

McCaw, Walter D. 1917. "An Introduction to the History of Medicine with Medical Chronology, Suggestions for Study and Bibliographic Data." Philadelphia: W. B. Saunders. https://archive.org/stream/introductiontohi00garruoft/introductiontohi00garruoft_djvu.txt. Accessed on April 19, 2017.

Merrill, Robin. 2016. *More Jesus Diet: More of God, Less of Me, Literally*. Royal Oak, MI: New Creation Publishing.

Miller, Karen Klahr. 2013. "Endocrine Effects of Anorexia Nervosa." *Endocrinology and Metabolism Clinics of North America*. 42(3): 515–528.

Molnar, Petra. 2011. "The Venus: Mother or Woman?" http://umanitoba.ca/publications/openjournal/index.php/ mb-anthro/article/viewFile/32/34. Accessed on April 9, 2017.

Morton, Richard. 1694. *Phthisiologia, or, a Treatise of Consumptions Wherein the Difference, Nature, Causes, Signs, and Cure of All Sorts of Consumptions Are Explained.* London: Sam. Smith and Benj. Walford. https://play .google.com/books/reader?id=_1_hlpTLRtYC&printsec= frontcover&output=reader&hl=en&pg=GBS.PA1. Accessed on April 12, 2017.

Norris, Mark L., et al. 2014. "Exploring Avoidant/Restrictive Food Intake Disorder in Eating Disordered Patients: A Descriptive Study." *International Journal of Eating Disorders.* 47(5): 495–499.

Ogden, Cynthia L., et al. 2016. "Prevalence of Obesity among Adults and Youth: United States, 2011–2014." NCHS Data Brief No. 219. November 2015. https:// www.cdc.gov/nchs/data/databriefs/db219.pdf. Accessed on April 6, 2017.

"Other Types of Eating Disorders." 2016. Eating Disorders. https://www.eatingdisorderfacts.com/. Accessed on November 27, 2018.

Papavramidou, Niki S., Spiros T. Papavramidis, and Helen Christopoulou-Aletra. 2004. "Galen on Obesity: Etiology, Effects, and Treatment." *World Journal of Surgery.* 28(6): 631–635.

Parry-Jones, Brenda. 1994. "Merycism or Rumination Disorder. A Historical Investigation and Current Assessment." *The British Journal of Psychiatry.* 165(3): 303–314.

Pearce, J. M. S. 2004. "Richard Morton: Origins of Anorexia Nervosa." *European Neurology.* 52(4): 191–192.

"The Physiology of Taste; or, Transcendental Gastronomy by Brillat-Savarin." 1826/2004. Project Gutenberg. http://www.gutenberg.org/ebooks/5434. Accessed on April 20, 2017.

Reda, Mario, and Giuseppe Sacco. 2001. "Anorexia and the Holiness of Saint Catherine of Siena." *Journal of Criminal Justice and Popular Culture.* 8(1): 37–47. http://www.albany.edu/scj/jcjpc/vol8is1/reda.html. Accessed on April 11, 2017.

Rogers, Oscar H. 1901. "Build as a Factor Influencing Longevity." https://books.google.com/books?id=EsUAA AAAYAAJ&pg=PA280&lpg=PA280&dq=%22Build+as+ a+Factor+Influencing+Longevity%22&source=bl&ots= cc7hoPdPul&sig=TgARv80I1y5uaSr0nOQyhnNItY0& hl=en&sa=X&ved=0ahUKEwiZp_2GkLbTAhVI_4MKH VPWBmEQ6AEIJTAB#v=onepage&q=twelfth&f=false. Accessed on April 21, 2017.

Rufe, Joan Brueggeman. 1994. "Early Christian Fasting: A Study of Creative Adaptation." Doctoral thesis, University of Virginia. http://phdtree.org/pdf/24923750-early-christian-fasting-a-study-of-creative-adaptation/. Accessed on April 10, 2017.

Russell, G. F. M. 1979. "Bulimia Nervosa: An Ominous Variant of Anorexia Nervosa." *Psychological Medicine.* 9(3): 429–448.

Sawbridge, D. T., and R. Fitzgerald. 2009. "'Lazy, Slothful and Indolent': Medical and Social Perceptions of Obesity in Europe to the Eighteenth Century." *Vesalius: Acta Internationales Historiae Medicinae.* 15(2): 59–70. http://www.vesalius.org.uk/images/issues/XV-2-2009.pdf. Accessed on April 17, 2017.

"Secrets of the Saints: The Forgotten Spiritual Power of Fasting." 2018. Church POP. https://churchpop.com/

2017/06/27/secrets-of-the-saints-the-forgotten-spiritual-power-of-fasting/. Accessed on November 27, 2018.

Sennertus, Daniel, N. Culpeper, and Abidiah Cole. 1664. *Practical Physick: The Fourth Book in Three Parts.* London: Peter Cole. https://books.google.com/books?id=G5BmAA AAcAAJ&pg=PA77&lpg=PA77&dq=practical+physick,+ the+fourth+book+galen&source=bl&ots=3t13O8v1Ic& sig=__LNGRd6uKqIZm8Dh_SCalPXqY8&hl=en&sa=X &ved=0ahUKEwjc6K6QhMXTAhXMy4MKHR39AEEQ 6AEIIzAA#v=onepage&q=practical%20physick%2C%20 the%20fourth%20book%20galen&f=false.

Shakespeare, William. ca. 1597. "The First Part of King Henry the Fourth." *The Complete Works of William Shakespeare.* http://shakespeare.mit.edu/1henryiv/full .html. Accessed on April 16, 2017.

Sheehan, H. L., and V. K. Summers. 1949. "The Syndrome of Hypopituitarism." *Quarterly Journal of Medicine.* 18(72): 319–378.

"Shiva: Matchmaker God." 2017. beliefnet. http://www .beliefnet.com/love-family/relationships/holidays/valentines-day/shiva-matchmaker-god.aspx. Accessed on April 10, 2017.

Sinkler, Wharton. 1898. "Rumination in Man." *The Journal of the American Medical Association.* 30(15): 834–837. https://books.google.com/books?id=DUkcAQAAMA AJ&pg=PA834&lpg=PA834&dq=%22rumination+in+ man%22+1894&source=bl&ots=8hVSfhQzMF&sig= CSnsMu7PXw4mLRD9J9SlevnG5C4&hl=en&sa=X& ved=0ahUKEwjG_77O3sXTAhWI7YMKHQBAC-oQ6AEIPDAF#v=onepage&q=%22rumination%20in% 20man%22%201894&f=true. Accessed on April 28, 2017.

Smart, Thomas. 1728. *A Discourse Concerning the Causes and Effects of Corpulency*, 2nd ed. London: J. Roberts. https:// books.google.com/books?id=nL9bAAAAcAAJ&pg=PA

20&lpg=PA20&dq=%22Discourse+Concerning+the+ Causes+and+Effects+of+Corpulency%22&source=bl&ots= P-svU1bg-e&sig=Oghya8VJHys9XjxPmSzphquCIy4&hl= en&sa=X&ved=0ahUKEwiij9zsjKzTAhUs0YMKHSjEDc cQ6AEISjAJ#v=onepage&q=no%20age&f=false. Accessed on April 19, 2017.

Smink, Frédérique R. E., Daphne van Hoeken, and Hans W. Hoek. 2012. "Epidemiology of Eating Disorders: Incidence, Prevalence and Mortality Rates." *Current Psychiatry Reports*. 14(4): 406–414.

Stunkard, Albert J. 1959. "Eating Patterns and Obesity." *Psychiatric Quarterly*. 33(2): 284–295.

Summers, V. K. 1947. "The Diagnosis and Treatment of Simmonds' Disease." *Postgraduate Medical Journal*. 23(263): 441–443.

Tasca, Cecillia, et al. 2012. "Women and Hysteria in the History of Mental Health." *Clinical Practice & Epidemiology in Mental Health*. 8(1): 110–119.

Tautges, Paul. 2007. *Delight in the Word Biblical Counsel for Everyday Issues: Gluttony, the Silent American Sin*. Enumclaw, WA: Pleasant Word.

T. E. C., Jr. 1969. "The Origin of the Word *Pica*." *Pediatrics*. 44(4): 548.

Thomas, J. J., L. R. Vartanian, and K. D. Brownell. 2009. "The Relationship between Eating Disorder Not Otherwise Specified (EDNOS) and Officially Recognized Eating Disorders: Meta-analysis and Implications for DSM." *Psychological Bulletin*. 135(3): 407–433.

Tripp, A. J., and N. E. Schmidt. 2013. "Analyzing Fertility and Attraction in the Paleolithic: The Venus Figurines." *Archaeology Ethnology and Anthropology of Eurasia*. 41(2): 54–60. https://www.researchgate.net/ publication/259523532_Analyzing_Fertility_and_ Attraction_in_the_Paleolithic_The_Venus_Figurines. Accessed on April 9, 2017.

Truswell, A. Stewart. 2013. "Medical History of Obesity." *Nutrition and Medicine.* 1(1): 1–25. https://opus .bibliothek.uni-wuerzburg.de/frontdoor/index/index/ docId/6707. Accessed on April 19, 2017.

Tubbs, R. D., et al. 2003. "Human Horns: A Historical Review and Clinical Correlation." *Neurosurgery.* 52(6): 1443–1447.

Van Wyhe, Cordula. 2017. "Did Rubens Make Big Beautiful?" BBC. http://www.bbc.co.uk/guides/zt6jq6f. Accessed on April 15, 2017.

Vigarello, Georges. 2013. *The Metamorphoses of Fat: A History of Obesity.* Trans. by C. Jon Delogu. New York: Columbia University Press.

Violatti, Cristian. 2013. "Vardhamana." Ancient History Encyclopedia. http://www.ancient.eu/Vardhamana/. Accessed on April 10, 2017.

White, Randall. 2006. "The Women of Brassempouy: A Century of Research and Interpretation." *Journal of Archaeological Method and Theory.* 13(4): 250–303. http:// blogimages.bloggen.be/evodisku/attach/166144.pdf. Accessed on April 10, 2017.

Whytt, Robert. 1765. *Observations on the Nature, Causes, and Cure of Those Disorders Which Have Been Commonly Called Nervous, Hypochondriac, or Hysteric.* London: T. Becket and P. A. De Honbt; Edinburgh: J. Balfour. https://archive.org/stream/observationsonna1767whyt/ observationsonna1767whyt_djvu.txt. Accessed on April 12, 2017.

Wilford, John Noble. 2009. "Full-Figured Statuette, 35,000 Years Old, Provides New Clues to How Art Evolved." *New York Times.* http://www.nytimes.com/2009/05/14/ science/14venus.html. Accessed on April 9, 2017.

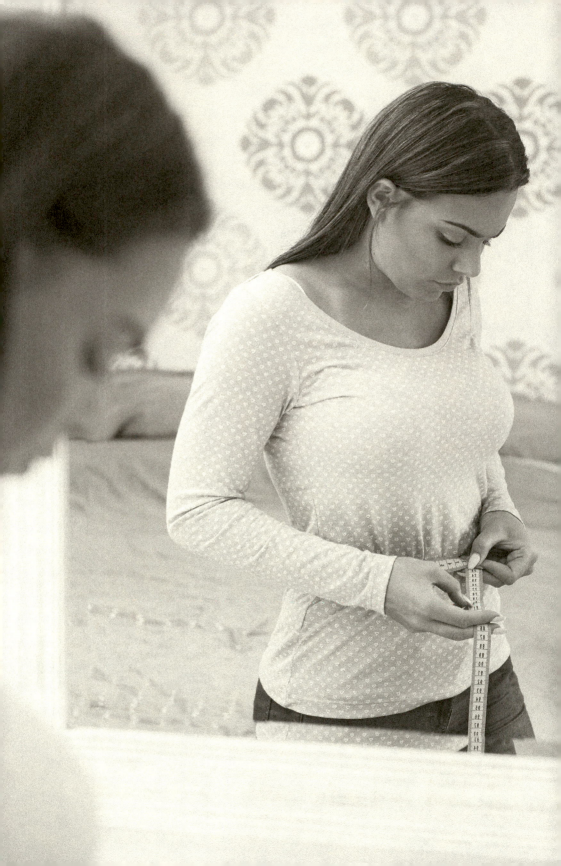

2 Problems, Issues, and Solutions

OK. So maybe I am a little bit overweight. Well, maybe a little bit more than "a little bit" overweight. But I have so many questions about my eating problems, such as the following:

- How do I really know if I'm *too* overweight or just "chubby" or "pleasantly plump"?
- Does it really matter all that much if I *am* overweight? I know lots of people who prefer someone who is fat.
- How did I develop this problem in the first place? Why can't I lose weight even when I try so hard to do so? Is my body somehow different from those of my friends who are of normal weight?
- What can I do about my eating problems? Is there a good diet, or a helpful book, or a smart counselor, or a reliable organization that I can contact?
- Suppose I do get my weight under control. How do I avoid gaining weight again in the future?
- I worry that my younger sister will develop some kind of eating problem. How can I help her to avoid the problem?

People with eating disorders often wonder about the diagnosis, effects, causes, treatment, prevention, and other questions of their condition. Each of these questions deserves an extended

---

An unhappy teenage girl measures her waist while looking in the mirror. (Ian Allenden/Dreamstime.com)

discussion. For each type of disorder, of course, the answer(s) to each question is somewhat different. This chapter reviews what is currently known about the answers to or guesses about each of these questions.

Diagnosing an Eating Disorder

Overweight and Obesity

Getting a general idea about a person's weight status is seldom a difficult task. Unlike high blood pressure, diabetes, or most other diseases, the first indication of an eating disorder can often be observed simply by visual examination; most people can tell if someone is grossly underweight or overweight. But specialists have a much more specific mechanism for diagnosing a person's weight status, the body mass index (BMI). To review, BMI is defined as a person's weight in kilograms divided by his or her height in meters. The formulas for BMI in the metric and English system are:

BMI = weight (kg)/height (m^2) or BMI = weight (pounds)/ height (in.^{2})

The U.S. National Institutes of Health uses the following standards (Table 2.1) to define the various types of weight in adults:

Table 2.1   BMI Standards

BMI	Classification
<18.5	Underweight
18.5 to <25.0	Normal
25.0 to <30.0	Overweight
>30.0	Obese

Source: Calculate Your Body Mass Index. 2018. National Heart, Lung, and Blood Institute. https://www.nhlbi.nih.gov/health/educational/lose_wt/BMI/bmicalc.htm. Accessed on November 27, 2018.

The category of "obese" is sometimes divided into other subcategories (Table 2.2).

Table 2.2   Categories of Obesity

BMI	Classification
30.0 to <35.0	Class 1
35.0 to <40.0	Class 2
>40.0	Class 3

Source: Calculate Your Body Mass Index. 2018. National Heart, Lung, and Blood Institute. https://www.nhlbi.nih.gov/health/educational/lose_wt/BMI/bmicalc.htm. Accessed on November 27, 2018.

All levels of obesity are thought to pose serious health problems, but Class 3 obesity is the most dangerous of the three subcategories. Individuals with Class 3 obesity are sometimes said to be *morbidly obese* because they are at high risk for a variety of health problems, such as diabetes, heart disease, sleep apnea, and osteoarthritis. (The term *morbid* means a condition causing or caused by a disease.) The same term is used for individuals with a BMI greater than 35.0 if they already have developed one or more of these conditions. The terms *severe* or *extreme* are also used to describe individuals with a BMI of Class 3.

Determining the BMI for a child or adolescent between the ages of 2 and 19 is a bit more complicated. Individuals in this age range grow at very different rates, so a person's age must be taken into account when calculating BMI. A simple calculation device is available for making this calculation, using the individual's age, height, and body weight. To see how such a calculator is used, see the "BMI Percentile Calculator for Child and Teen" at https://nccd.cdc.gov/dnpabmi/calculator.aspx. If you are within this age range, you can enter your own birthdate, weight, and height and find your own BMI. Using this calculator will also tell you whether you would be classified as underweight, normal, overweight, or obese.

Other Eating Disorders

Very strict criteria for diagnosing anorexia, bulimia, binge eating disorder, and other eating disorders are provided in the latest edition of the *Diagnostic and Statistical Manual of Mental Disorders*, currently *DSM-V*. For example, the criteria for a diagnosis of anorexia nervosa in *DSM-V* include an energy intake that is inadequate to meet the normal requirements for a person of his or her age, sex, and physical health; an intense fear of gaining weight; and undue concerns about one's body shape or the way in which his or her weight is distributed (Anorexia Nervosa 2015). Any person examined by a health-care worker who appears to have the distinctive characteristics of one of these eating disorders is usually seen by a psychiatrist or other trained medical worker, who then uses the complete set of criteria for making a final diagnosis of the patient's condition.

But a number of signs are available by which a person can be judged at risk for an eating disorder. The most obvious signs are ones that an observer can easily pick out, such as an obvious refusal to eat, a significant loss in weight, or visits to the bathroom for long periods of time after a meal. But a number of more subtle signs are also available. Some of the signs of anorexia that have been suggested by professionals in the field include the following:

- A denial that one is hungry
- Exhibiting an unusual selectivity for the kinds of foods one eats
- Unusual attention to the caloric value of foods or the number of calories one consumes in a day
- Preparing especially elaborate meals for family or friends, in which the individual himself or herself does not take part
- Development of certain ritualized eating habits, such as moving one's food about on the plate
- Unusual use of laxatives or purgatives
- Use of excuses to avoid meals or other occasions for eating
- Increased isolation from families and friends

- Mood changes, such as demonstrations of anxiety or depression
- Reduced ability to get along with others
- Wearing of heavy coats or other bulky types of clothing
- Unusual tiredness and fatigue
- Unusual interest and involvement in exercise
- Fidgeting and other forms of nervousness
- For women, changes in menstrual periods
- Pale skin and lusterless hair

(Many Internet sites provide suggestions such as these. See, e.g., Anorexia Nervosa 2015; Home/Learn by Eating Disorder 2016; Understanding the Warning Signs 2015.)

One of the most important cautions involved with a list of this kind, however, is that no one behavior, or combination of behaviors, definitely indicates the presence of an eating disorder. Any number of reasons may explain a person's demonstrating a behavior that has nothing to do with one's eating desires. No ordinary person should assume the role of a professional health-care worker in diagnosing eating disorders. Some ongoing combination of these signs may, however, suggest that a person may need a friend to talk to, a counselor to see, a book to read, or some other assistance with the problems in his or her life.

Signs and symptoms for other eating disorders are different from those of anorexia. But, like anorexia, they generally have very specific symptoms as defined by *DSM-V* (see Chapter 1 for more details on these DSM symptoms). Other eating disorders also have distinctive signs, *warning signs*, less specific than those outlined by *DSM-V*, but still very suggestive of possible eating problem. For example, typical signs for bulimia tend to be very different from those of anorexia because they reflect the thoughts and feelings of someone whose goal is to overeat, rather than undereat, before purging or otherwise eliminating the food just ingested. Some of the warning signs of bulimia include the following:

- Binge eating occurs commonly.
- Purging behavior is indicated by frequent trips to the bathroom after ingesting a meal.
- May steal and hoard food for consumption at a later time.
- May show signs of body damage as a result of purging, such as discolored teeth or sores around the mouth or on the hands.
- Has a tendency to diet frequently.
- May have a tendency to check his or her appearance in a mirror to make sure his or her body appearance is "up to par."
- Physical signs, such as dizziness, fainting, vacillating weight patterns, dry skin, fine hair, tooth problems, and difficulties in concentrating (Bulimia Nervosa 2017; Eating Disorders 2017; The Effects of Bulimia on the Body 2017; Home/ Learn by Eating Disorder 2016).

Binge eating disorder has some features in common with bulimia nervosa in that a person ingests much more food than is necessary for one's nutritional needs, generally eating long after he or she is satiated ("full"). It also has some subtle signs and symptoms similar to those of bulimia, such as preferring to eat alone, dieting, and feeling guilt about one's eating habits. It differs from bulimia, however, in that gorging is not followed by purging or other forms of evacuation. Binge eating is also not accompanied by most of the other signs of either anorexia or bulimia (Ekern 2017).

For some types of eating disorders, the clinical (*DSM-V*) signs and symptoms are so clear that there may not be much question as to what type of problem a person is suffering from. For example, a child who continually eats chips of paint that have flaked off a wall is almost certainly suffering from pica. Other abnormal eating problems may also be easy to discern and thus suggest a diagnosis of pica. The same might be said for ruminant disorder and orthorexia, in which an unusual eating pattern is fairly easy to observe. In a group eating situation, for example, a person who regurgitates and then re-ingests his or her food is difficult to miss. And someone who is obsessive about the color, taste, origin, nutritional value, or other feature of a food rather clearly suggests that he or she is dealing with orthorexia (Koven and Abry 2015).

Still, additional subtle signs of these conditions may be observed. For example, in the case of rumination disorder, a person may display signs such as abdominal pain, constipation, nausea, diarrhea, bloating, inability to produce feces, and weight loss. The problem is that these signs are not very characteristic of ruminant disorder exclusively but are associated with a rather wide variety of other disorders. Both clinicians and everyday observers, then, are likely to rely on more direct evidence, such as actual observance of the behavior (Attri et al. 2008; Bhandari 2016).

The symptoms of avoidant/restrictive food intake disorder (ARFID) are somewhat similar to those of orthorexia, in that they involve "picky" eating by an individual. In fact, an older term for ARFID, selective eating disorder, highlights this characteristic of the condition. Some of the other signs that might suggest a person is suffering from ARFID include a person's reluctance to eat at all, or at least certain foods at certain times of the day in certain settings; a preference for eating alone; a slow pace of eating when one does agree to have a meal; irrational fears of choking or vomiting; a failure to gain weight for a person of the subject's age and gender, or even a loss of weight in such a case; or a general failure to mature physically for the person's age and gender (Grewal and Lieberman 2016; Warning Signs and Symptoms [for ARFID] 2016; Zickgraf, Franklin, and Rozin 2016).

As described in Chapter 1, the category of other specified feeding and eating disorders (OSFED) is new to *DSM-V*, replacing another term, eating disorder not otherwise specified

(EDNOS). The category includes any and all eating disorders that are not otherwise listed in one of the other categories listed earlier. Because it covers such a wide range of conditions, the signs and symptoms for OSFED are extensive and broad. They include such mental and physical signs and symptoms as the following:

- Weight changes that cannot be explained by other factors
- Changes in menstrual patterns for females and interest in sexual activities among males
- An increased tendency to develop diseases, as an indication of a compromised immune system
- Indications of frequent vomiting, such as damage to the teeth, the mouth, and regions around the mouth, as well as on the hands and arms
- Lack of physical stability, as reflected in dizziness and nausea
- An abnormal concern about eating meals, certain foods, or eating patterns
- Concerns about one's body image
- Anxiety about eating with others
- General lack of confidence and loss of self-esteem, in general (Other Specified Feeding or Eating Disorders [OSFED] 2017; What Is OSFED? 2017)

(As is the case with all other eating disorders, many of these symptoms are quite nonspecific and may be caused by physical and/or mental problems other than an eating disorder. The layperson should never "rush to judgment" about the possibility of a family member or friend's likelihood of having developed an eating disorder. Such diagnoses can be made only by trained personnel, such as a psychiatrist or other medical doctor.)

Effects of Eating Disorders

All eating disorders disrupt, in one way or another, a person's normal eating patterns. That disruption is based on the fact that a person ingests too much or not enough of the substances one needs to grow, maintain good health, and avoid disease. These effects may begin to show up soon after one begins to alter one's eating habit. But they also tend to accumulate and worsen over time with serious, sometimes irreversible, effects on the body and mind. For all forms of eating disorders, the ultimate long-term effect may be death.

Anorexia

Most of the short-term effects of anorexia are changes in the body and mind that can be detected by an outside observer as a warning sign for the condition. They may include changes such as unexplained weight loss; changes in one's bowel movements (usually constipation); dehydration from loss of water through vomiting; unusual fatigue; a tendency toward dizziness, confusion, and/or fainting; abnormally dry skin and hair; insomnia; and a poor overall health condition accompanied by an increased risk for infectious diseases.

All of these conditions are, of course, of concern to an individual with anorexia, his or her family and friends, and the person's health-care provider. Without early treatment, this and other eating disorders soon begin to cause more long-term and more serious physical and mental health problems. These changes are generally of considerably more importance for children and adolescents than for their older counterparts. Adolescence, in particular, is a period of rapid growth on body systems. According to some studies, a person experiences about a quarter of his or her adult height gain during adolescence, about half of his or her gain in adult weight, and development of the reproductive system that ensures a healthy and normal biological mechanism for the ability to produce new individuals at a later point in life. All of these changes require an adequate input of carbohydrates, protein, fats, vitamins and minerals, and other nutrients, a condition that is virtually impossible for anyone struggling with anorexia (Sidiropoulos 2007).

Generally, the first long-term effect observed for anorexia is reduced formation of bony material, or actual loss of bone mass. After puberty, the rate of bone growth in the normal boy or girl is about 8 percent per year. This growth occurs when bone-making cells known as *osteocytes* begin the process of changing fibrous material in a child into bone. Anorexia interrupts this stage of development by slowing down or inhibiting the action of osteocytes, reducing the rate at which new bone growth occurs. This effect results in the failure of an individual's body to develop what would otherwise be its normal height and body structure. A second effect occurs when the lack of nutrients that occurs with anorexia causes the system that repairs existing bone material to fail, resulting in an increased risk for bone fractures (Adkins 2017; Misra and Klibanski 2014; What People with Anorexia Nervosa Need to Know about Osteoporosis 2016).

Another long-term effect of anorexia involves the heart and circulatory system. A failure of the body to receive adequate amounts of the nutrients it needs to function properly has a variety of effects on the heart and circulatory system. Among the most common of these effects is a condition known as *bradycardia*, a situation in which a person's heartbeat slows down below normal, typically defined as less than 60 beats a minute. Bradycardia results in the heart's reduced efficiency in moving blood through the circulatory system, which can result in feelings of exhaustion and tiredness that are typical of anorexia. Bradycardia is observed in nearly all (95 percent) of people with anorexia (Yahalom et al. 2013).

Bradycardia and the loss of nutrients may also have other effects on the heart, such as structural changes in the heart muscle itself. These changes may result in loss of muscle mass in the heart, thereby reducing its ability to push blood through the heart and the body. Another effect is the loss of contractility in the heart, the ability of the heart muscle to exert sufficient pressure to drive blood through the circulatory system. One general effect of these changes in the heart is sudden death, an event that may occur before an individual even realizes that his or her heart has been damaged by anorexia. The loss of cardiac contractivity is also a consequence of the development of electrolyte imbalance in the body as a result of poor nutrition. Electrolyte imbalance refers to a change in the normal and necessary composition of sodium, potassium, chloride, calcium, and other ions in the body that control many of its basic functions. Probably the best-known example of death from anorexia caused by these changes was that of popular signer Karen Carpenter, who died in 1983 at the age of 32 from anorexia-related causes. During the last year of her life, in fact, she complained about some of the heart-related symptoms described here (Schmidt 2010; also see Garrido and Lobera 2012; Sachs et al. 2016; Yahalom et al. 2013; for other physiological effects of anorexia, see Meczekalski, Podfigurna-Stopa, and Katulski 2013; Mehler and Brown 2015; Sidiropoulos 2007).

The short- and long-term effects of anorexia go far beyond physical changes and issues. Anorexia, after all, like all eating disorders, is fundamentally a mental health problem with physical consequences. It should hardly be surprising, then, that changes in one's eating patterns always affect the way one thinks about and feels about other people and the world around that person. Furthermore, it is worthy of note that psychological issues can be both the cause of eating disorders like anorexia and the end results of those conditions (but more about this later in this chapter).

One of the most common emotions caused by anorexia is depression. This relationship might be thought of as a "chicken and egg" issue: which comes first, depression, which leads to an eating disorder, or an eating disorder, which then leads to depression? It's possible that both patterns may exist in any one example of the disorder. In any case, current evidence now suggests that the mental state (depression) may actually be a result of changes in the brain that occur as a result of poor eating habits. The condition may manifest itself as simply feeling sad and estranged from friends and family, as a tendency to become angry and unhappy with other people's actions, or as a desire to be alone so as not to have to interact with others. Depression may also be associated with feelings of low esteem that often accompany anorexia. Depression may also express itself in the form of reduced interest in sexual activities and a tendency toward self-mutilation, in the form of cutting or burning one's body. Again, at least some or all of most, if not all, of these mental changes can now be traced to specific changes in the brain, often a change in hormone production and action because of inadequate nutrition (Barbarich, Kaye, and Jimerson 2003; Eating Disorders—The Physical and Psychological Consequences of Eating Disorders 2017; Jade 2012).

Other consequences of anorexia include feelings of shame, poor self-worth, anxiety, and guilt about one's condition. Anorexia may also lead to the development of obsessive-compulsive disorder (OCD). OCD is a type of anxiety in which a person tends to repeat the same idea, feeling, sensation, thought, or behavior over and over again (a *compulsion*). A common method of dealing with OCD is for a person to develop a rigorous schedule for one or more activities in one's life, such as rechecking over and over again whether a door is locked or the stove is turned off; saying, counting, or behaving the same action many times over; focusing on one's cleanliness by repeatedly laundering clothes and other items even when they do not need to be; making sure all the items in one's life are always in the proper place; and accumulating objects and materials for which there is almost certainly no future use (The Effects of Starvation on Behavior: Implications for Dieting and Eating Disorders 2015).

The appearance of a mental disorder in association with anorexia (and other eating disorders) illustrates a condition known as *comorbidity*. Comorbidity is the occurrence of two or more physical and/or mental conditions at the same time. For example, individuals who become anorexic may eventually develop a number of other conditions, such as depression, anxiety, and/or OCD (e.g., Bühren et al. 2014; Kaye et al. 2004; Mascolo et al. 2017; Padez-Vieira and Afonso 2016).

Bulimia

As with anorexia, a host of physical and psychological problems may be associated with bulimia, most of which are related to emesis, the process of vomiting that is an integral part of bulimia. One of the most characteristic of these signs is a condition known as *Russell's sign*, which consists of scarring on the hands and fingers that develops as a result of a person's inserting his or hand into the mouth to induce vomiting (Daluiski, Rahbar, and Meals 1997). A number of other dermatological signs may be present in the bulimic patient, including nail fragility; abnormal growth of hair on the body (Ambras syndrome; hypertrichosis lanuginosa); inflammation, drying, and cracking of the lips (cheilosis); loss of hair (alopecia); abnormally dry skin (xerosis); and itchiness of the skin (pruritis) (Renata 2013, passim; for a good general overview of the physical effects of bulimia, see Brown 2017).

Emesis may also have significant effects on a person's teeth and gums. The acidic character of the vomitus (vomited material) attacks tooth enamel and may lead to a number of dental problems, including caries (tooth decay), increased sensitivity of the teeth, reduction in production of saliva, dry mouth, and periodontal disease (Dynesen et al. 2008; Valena and Young 2002; vomitus typically has a pH [acidity] of about 0.8, equivalent to the strongest of mineral acids, such as hydrochloric acid).

Additional effects of bulimia extend to the throat and gastrointestinal system. Again, the strongly acidic character of swallowed vomitus may cause damage to the esophagus and the lining of the stomach and intestines. Some of the specific complaints arising from this condition are gastroesophageal reflux, esophagitis (inflammation of the esophagus), esophageal cancer, stomach ulcers, stomach pain, and constipation and irregular bowel movements and/or diarrhea (Denholm and Jankowski 2011; Lionetti et al. 2011). Other disorders may develop as a result of a bulimic's use of laxatives or diuretics to discharge excess foods. The most important effect of these materials is an alteration in the balance of electrolytes in the body. Electrolytes such as ions of sodium, potassium, calcium, chloride, and bicarbonate exert significant control over a number of critical biological functions. Changes in the balance of electrolytes, then, can in and of themselves produce a wide variety of gastrointestinal and other effects (Bell 2015; Zepf 2004).

Binge Eating Disorder

The primary way in which binge eating disorder differs from bulimia is that the former practice results in a person's continually gaining weight; most of the food he or she eats is stored in the body. The effects that one sees from binge eating, then, are similar to those for obesity. Specifically, a binge eater can expect to experience increased risk for heart disease, type 2 diabetes, arthritis, some forms of cancer, gout, irritable bowel syndrome, gallbladder disease, digestive problems, muscle pain, and sleep apnea (Binge Eating Disorder 2017; Goldberg 2017).

As with other eating disorders, binge eating is accompanied by a number of mental, emotional, and psychological problems. A person is likely to feel "trapped" by his or her eating disorder, lacking an understanding and/or desire to return to normal eating habits. This attitude may lead to feelings of anger, anxiety, depression, moodiness, guilt, and poor self-worth. At that point, it's easy to withdraw from one's family and friends and to begin avoiding one's usual social activities, leading to additional feelings of separation and loneliness.

Other Eating Disorders

Each of the other eating disorders discussed in this book has its own set of short- and long-term consequences.

Pica

Long-term consequences of pica eating disorder depend almost entirely on the material a person chooses to eat. Anyone who ingests paint chips, for example, is at risk for toxic materials that may be present in the paint, most commonly compounds of lead. Someone who eats dirt, cigarette ashes, or other inorganic materials runs the risk of nutrient deficiencies because he or she is taking in food with no nutritional value. Some otherwise harmless materials may also contain bacteria, viruses, molds, or other disease-causing agents. The ingestion of unsuitable materials, such as dirt and sand, may also result in physical problems, such as damage to the intestinal lining and/ or abdominal pain (Stiegler 2005).

Ruminant Disorder

Since ruminant disorder is somewhat related to bulimia because of the emesis involved, one might expect the short- and long-term consequences of the two conditions to be similar. Among the events that are often listed as complications of ruminant disorder are malnutrition, lowered resistance to infections and diseases, failure to grow and thrive, weight loss, stomach diseases such as ulcers, dehydration, halitosis, tooth decay, respiratory problems such as pneumonia, and choking. Under some circumstances, the condition may also lead to a person's death (Bhandari 2016; Malcolm et al. 1997).

Orthorexia

Orthorexia is one of the least understood of all eating disorders. The condition was first named in 1997 by California physician Steven Bratman, Some dispute still exists as to its classification as a discrete eating disorder. As data accumulate, however, one thing is clear: people who conscientiously set out to eat the most healthful diet they can imagine may put themselves at risk for life-threatening, long-term consequences. The problem is that such individuals may choose a very specific set of foods to eat, thus increasing the likelihood of their missing out on other foods that may provide essential nutrients. This reasoning explains some of the most common complications that may arise from an orthorexic diet: a host of possible nutrient deficiencies (e.g., anemia); general malnutrition; a less effective immune system; kidney problems, including kidney failure; osteoporosis; heart disease; and infertility. As with all other types of eating disorders, other complications may involve mental, emotional, or psychological issues, such as anxiety, feelings of stress, low feelings of self-worth, general emotional instability, social isolation, and OCD (Bratman 2017).

Other Eating Disorders

The short- and long-term consequences of both ARFID and EDNOS cannot so easily be summarized. In the case of ARFID, the formal diagnosis is fairly new, and relatively little research has been conducted on the condition. The general consensus appears to be that the long-term effects of ARFID are similar to those of anorexia nervosa because the behaviors associated with both conditions are very similar. The most important difference between the two is the role of intention. That is, individuals with anorexia nervosa want and plan to lose weight, while those with ARFID lack that motivation; the condition arises and is maintained for other, still not clearly understood reasons (Nicely et al. 2014).

The situation with EDNOS is somewhat different. That category of eating disorders is somewhat broad and still not well studied or understood. It includes subcategories of conditions that are similar to other eating disorders, such as atypical anorexia nervosa, bulimia nervosa of low frequency and/or duration, binge eating disorder of low frequency and/or duration, purging disorder, and night-eating syndrome. The long-term effects of these various subcategories tend to be similar to those with which they are associated (e.g., atypical anorexia nervosa with anorexia nervosa). In some ways, this fact creates problems for therapists and others interested in eating disorders. As some authorities have pointed out, the very name suggests that EDNOS may be a less serious type of eating disorder, with less serious consequences than anorexia, bulimia, or other conditions. As a result, the condition may not be diagnosed or treated as conscientiously as are other eating disorders (Battiste and Effron 2012; EDNOS: The Silent Killer 2013).

Overweight and Obesity

The physical and emotional effects of overweight and obesity have now been studied in considerable detail. Evidence now suggests that a number of conditions may be caused by weight issues, including body pain and difficulty with physical functioning; various types of cancer, including breast, colon, endometrial, gallbladder, kidney, and liver; coronary heart disease; dyslipidemia (high LDL cholesterol, low HDL cholesterol, or high levels of triglycerides); gallbladder disease; hypertension (high blood pressure), metabolic syndrome; osteoarthritis (loss of bone and cartilage in joints); sleep apnea and other breathing problems; stroke; and type 2 diabetes (Pi-Sunyer 2015). In addition, overweight and obesity have been implicated in a number of mental disorders, such as anxiety, clinical depression, distorted body image, low self-esteem, other mood disorders, risk for eating disorders, and substance abuse. All of these effects may lead to a generally depressed quality of life for overweight and obese individuals, as well as a significantly increased mortality. Experimental evidence for these correlations tends, however, to be less sound than are those for physical effects (Magallares and Pais-Ribeiro 2014).

Causes of Eating Disorders

Arguably the single most important question about eating disorders focuses on how they are caused. If the cause of an eating disorder is known, that information contributes to an under-standing of how that disorder can be diagnosed, what signs and symptoms it is likely to evoke, what short- and long-term consequences can be expected, and how the condition can be prevented and treated. Too little is known for sure about each of the specific eating disorders, and some dispute remains as to which possible cause is most important and how it exerts its effects on an individual. The following sections review some of the current knowledge and hypotheses about the causes of the specific eating disorders.

Risk Factors

One of the first steps in identifying the causes of eating disor-ders is to discover what risk factors, if any, may be associated with a condition. A *risk factor* is a circumstance that increases the likelihood that an individual will develop some type of ad-verse health event in his or her life. As an example, a risk factor for diabetes is obesity. That statement means that individuals who are obese are at a greater risk for developing diabetes than are those who are less heavy.

Notice that risk factors do not unquestionably identify the *causes* of a disease or disorder. As an example, suppose that re-searchers find out that the children of parents with Narbovian heritage (a fictitious country) have a greater number of dental caries (cavities) than do children whose parents have a differ-ent heritage. One can say, then, that Narbovian heritage is a risk factor for dental caries. That statement does not mean that Narbovian heritage causes dental caries, only that there is a sta-tistical connection between the two variables. An alternative explanation might be that some third factor, such as traditional eating patterns that include a great deal of sugar in the case of Narbovians, is responsible for the onset of dental caries. Nor does the risk statement say that there is not necessarily any-thing wrong about individuals who have a risk factor for some type of disease or disorder. In many cases, an individual may be born with that risk factor. To mention an absurd example, a risk factor for miscarriages is being a woman. That is, only women can become pregnant, so the risk factor for a man's having a miscarriage is zero.

Therefore, what is the benefit of knowing the risk factors for some disease or condition, such as an eating disorder? For one thing, having that information may help in programs of prevention for a disorder. If one knows, for example, that the risk of developing anorexia is increased by exposure to unsuitable media presentations of the "ideal" body type, then a variety of actions can be taken to reduce the chance that individuals will develop anorexia. Efforts can be made to educate children, adolescents, and adults about the effects of such media presentations, and/or political, legal, social, or other actions can be taken against media organizations that perpetuate such ideal images.

Another useful aspect of risk factors is that they provide researchers with leads as to possible causes for a disease or disorder. Returning to the Narbovian example, knowing that a person's ethnic, racial, or other heritage increases one's risk for dental caries, a researcher might decide to see if there is any cause-and-effect relationship, allowing him or her to obtain that valuable information as to what it is in a person's life that causes that person to develop anorexia, bulimia, or some other eating disorder.

Given that background, it is possible to list a number of risk factors that researchers have identified as increasing one's likelihood of developing some type of eating disorder. Those risk factors fall into a few general categories, among the most important of which are genetic ("Was I born with a predisposition for anorexia?"), psychological ("Has something altered my way of thinking and feeling about food that has caused my bulimia?"), and social ("Are there forces in the world around me that have caused the development of my binge eating disorder?"). Some of the risk factors for eating disorders that have been recognized are the following:

- Family relationships: Individuals who have a close relative who has struggled with an eating disorder or who has had a mental illness are more likely to develop an eating disorder themselves.

- Age: Eating disorders may occur at any point in a person's life. But just statistically, young adults and those in their twenties are more likely to develop such conditions than are those who are very young or more than 30 years (Allen et al. 2014; Bulik 2002).

- Being female: Although eating disorders may affect both males and females, they tend to occur far more commonly among girls and women than among boys and men (Prevalence in Men 2017).

- Psychological issues: Individuals with any one of a variety of psychological problems—such as low self-esteem, anxiety, depression, feelings of anxiety, obsessive-compulsive behavior, sense of perfectionism, and inflexibility—are at risk for eating disorders (Tomba et al. 2014).

- Cultural factors: Many forces in the world around us tend to promote ideal images for males and females, such as advertising, popular entertainment, and sports figures. The more seriously a person takes these messages, the more likely he or she will depend on an eating disorder (e.g., Stice and Whitenton 2002).

- Sexual orientation: Research suggests that members of the LGBTQ community are at greater risk for eating disorders than are their heterosexual counterparts. One reason suggested for this pattern is the stress felt by individuals whose sexual norm is different from that of the general population (Eating Disorders in LGBT Populations 2017).

- Extracurricular activities: Somewhat surprisingly, involvement in extracurricular activities, such as sports and theatrical productions, may place a person at risk for eating disorders. The reason for this association is that coaches and teachers may, intentionally or accidentally, pressure boys and girls/young men and women to strive for body structures that are more suitable for the activities in which they are involved (Curie 2010; Francisco, Alarcáo, and Narciso 2012).

- Changes in one's life: Experts in the field believe that significant changes in one's life—such as a parental breakup, moving to a new city and/or school, taking on a new job or losing an old one, or undergoing a health crisis—places one at risk for an eating disorder. One explanation for the phenomenon is that such changes may lead to many of the feelings and emotion, such as stress and uncertainty, that themselves are risk factors for eating disorders (Bachar et al. 2008).

- Dieting: Studies have shown that individuals who begin dieting, for example, in the desire simply to lose weight, may then continue their efforts by adopting some form of eating disorder. This problem is compounded by the fact that about two-thirds of all young adults who diet also increase their activity level by exercising, a combination that can lead to rapid and unhealthy weight loss (Stice and Burger 2015).

(For some general references on risk factors for loss-of-weight eating disorders, see Hinney et al. 2006; Magallares 2013; Sansone and Sansone 2010; Striegel-Moore and Bulk 2007.)

Many of the risk factors for loss-of-weight eating disorders, such as anorexia and bulimia, also apply to problems of overweight and obesity. However, some additional risk factors for these conditions have also been identified. They include the following:

- Unhealthy eating habits, which includes consuming foods high in sugar and foods containing too many saturated and trans fats and, in general, consuming more calories than one actually needs to lead a healthy lifestyle.

- Lack of exercise and other types of physical activities, which reduces the number of calories expended compared to the number of calories included in one's diet.

- Lack of an adequate amount of sleep, which has been shown to be correlated with a gain in weight.

- Certain medications and medical conditions my place one at risk for obesity. Included in this list are certain types of antidepressants, antiseizure medications, diabetes medications, antipsychotic medications, steroids, and beta blockers, as well as conditions such as Prader-Willi syndrome and Cushing's syndrome.

- Smoking cessation can also lead to weight gain, although the health benefits of stopping smoking are probably greater overall than the risks posed by tobacco itself (Diseases and Conditions: Obesity. Risk Factors 2017; Segel 2010).

Etiology of Eating Disorders

Scholars have proposed a wide variety of hypotheses about the cause(s) of eating disorders for hundreds of years. These hypotheses date back at least to the Middle Ages. More recently, researchers have carried out an untold number of scientific studies on this issue. Although a considerable amount of information has resulted from these studies, much uncertainty remains, and many questions have yet to be answered about the etiology of eating disorders.

For most of the early history of eating disorders (i.e., until about the beginning of the nineteenth century), common explanations for the existence of eating disorders were based primarily in theology. Individuals who practiced self-starvation were thought to be possessed by one of two very contrary forces, either a strong demonic influence or a strong drive for salvation (Bemporad 1997; Dell'Osso et al. 2016). Such explanations gradually lost their influence over the next two centuries but have not disappeared completely today. In an interview telecast in May 2015, for example, the famous evangelist Pat

Robertson declared that eating disorders might be thought of as "a demonic possession thing" (Blue 2015; also see Symptoms of Demonic Bondage 2017; Throckmorton 2016). Very few reputable scholars today, however, give much credence to this theory.

Current thinking suggests that some factor or combination of factors may explain the etiology of more than one type of eating disorder. Some forces, for example, can be at work in the development of anorexia, bulimia, ARFID, and EDNOS. In other cases, more specific factors can be identified in the etiology of specific disorders, such as binge eating, pica, and orthorexia. Modern causal theories of anorexia and bulimia specifically tend to fall into one of three (or some combination of) major categories: psychological, environmental, and biological. (Possibly the best currently available reference on this topic is Polivy and Herman 2002. Although somewhat outdated, this work provides useful information on virtually all topics discussed later.)

Psychological Factors

Some of the characteristics of an individual's personal psychology that may predispose a person toward anorexia, bulimia, or similar weight-loss eating disorders include a drive for perfection in one's appearance; a more general concern about one's weight; low self-esteem and lack of confidence; OCD; high standards for one's personal achievements; a desire to gain control over one's life; high levels of strife; personal loss, as in the death of a parent or close friend; a tendency to withdraw from or avoid social interactions; a preoccupation with order and neatness in one's life; and rigid thinking about approaching life's everyday problems.

One of the most commonly observed psychological causes of anorexia and bulimia is perfectionism, the striving for a body image or personality traits that will meet some exterior standard, such as the representation of an ideal individual established by outside standards. A number of studies have confirmed the role of perfectionism in the development of eating disorders. For example, a 2003 study of 70 women who had been diagnosed with anorexia found that about 10 percent of the subjects claimed that their own efforts at achieving perfection were responsible for their eating disorders (Tozzi et al. 2003, 149, table 3). These results were obtained in interviews in which subjects gave their own versions of the causes of their eating disorders. In another study, 322 women subjects of a study were asked to take psychological tests to determine the causes of their anorexia. In this experiment, the anorexic women scored significantly higher on a test of perfectionism than did a non-anorexic control group. The authors of the study concluded that "the present results support the notion that perfectionism is a prominent feature of the personality background of individuals affected with anorexia nervosa" (Halmi et al. 2000, 1803). A somewhat different perspective on the issue can be found in an eight-year study of males and females in Sweden who had been anorexic at the time the study began and later no longer displayed symptoms of their condition. When asked what they believed was the cause of their original condition, participants provided answers of the type: "I want to be perfect; did not feel good, I've also placed very high expectations on myself about achievement. I've placed these demands on myself" (Nilsson et al. 2007, 129).

Any number of studies dating back more than three decades have also identified low self-esteem as a contributing factor to the development of eating disorders. The term *self-esteem* refers to the way a person regards his or her physical, mental, emotional, and other personal features. It is characterized by feelings of unworthiness, incompetence, unattractiveness, inability to deal with social situations, and general dissatisfaction with one's own life. For example, one study of 200 women and girls between the ages of 13 and 19 who had been diagnosed with an eating disorder confirmed the results of earlier studies, showing that individuals with low self-esteem were more likely to have developed eating disorders than those in a control group. The results leading to this conclusion were based on interviews with the women and girls and the results of three different written measures of self-esteem. The study further found that the severity of an individual's problems was related to the degree of her self-esteem, with those having lower self-confidence showing greater eating disorders problems (Rutsztein, Scappatura, and Murawski 2014). In one of the studies cited earlier, a person with anorexia described this issue in very specific terms. "I have low self-confidence and self-esteem," she told in an interview, "so I wanted to hurt myself." She then explained that she "let myself get hungry so it hurt. It felt good" (Nilsson et al. 2007, 130; for a summary on current research on eating disorders and self-esteem, see Welch and Ghaderi 2012).

Individuals with eating disorders also report that self-control is a factor in the development of their anorexia, bulimia, or other condition. The term *self-control* has been defined as "the ability to override or change individuals' inner responses, disrupt unwanted behavioral tendencies (such as impulses) and abstain from acting on them" (Tangney, Baumeister, and Boone 2004). Individuals, often children and adolescents, may descend into an emotional state in which they feel they have no control over their lives. They may, for example, have domineering parents, a difficult living arrangement, or a school experience in which they feel that all the important decisions in their lives are being made by someone else, with little or no hope that that situation will change. But the one thing such individuals *can* control is their eating habits. Studies have now shown that by *choosing* how, when, what, and whether to eat, persons can feel some control over at least one aspect of their lives. And with that feeling, they may also develop the hope that they can develop control also in other parts of their life. An eating disorder, in such a case, becomes a strengthening and empowering part of one's life (Sassaroli, Gallucci, and Ruggiero. 2008).

The connection between control and eating disorders has now been confirmed by a number of studies. The relationship apparently is not, however, as straightforward as it may seem. In one study of the phenomenon, for example, researchers found that a group of women with either anorexia or bulimia *did* report having low confidence with regard to control issues, but, somewhat surprisingly, they also expressed very little desire to change that condition. That finding does raise some questions about the way in which control issues actually affect a person's choice to alter his or her eating habits (Tiggemann and Raven 1998).

Eating disorders have also been found to develop among individuals with any one of a variety of anxiety disorders. An *anxiety disorder* is a mental condition characterized by serious concerns about future events. One type of anxiety disorders is OCD, in which a person attempts to find ways of dealing with his or her anxiety. The individual may decide that performing certain specific actions over and over again in a ritualized way may prevent the occurrence of some disruptive or unknown event or events in the future. OCD gets its name from the fact that a person develops certain fixed ideas (concerns) about a future event, an *obsession*, about such an event, and attempts to prevent or ameliorate such an event by specified actions, a *compulsion*.

There now exists a substantial amount of evidence that a person with OCD stands a greater chance of developing an eating disorder than does someone without OCD. The significance of that effect, however, is somewhat in question. Researchers have reported a likelihood that a person with OCD will later develop an eating disorder at anywhere from 11 to 86 percent of the time. One reason for this vast range of results is probably that the pool of individuals who have or have had both OCD and eating disorders is relatively small. In spite of this fact, however, there now appears to be no doubt that the occurrence of an anxiety disorder, especially OCD, is one cause for the development of an eating disorder (Buckner, Silgado, and Lewinsohn 2010; Micali et al. 2011).

Environmental Factors

The term *environmental factors* in this discussion refers to all forces outside the body of a person dealing with an eating disorder. These factors include the family, peer pressure, patterns of being bullied, societal expectations and demands, mass media, and personal trauma. In the real world, it is often difficult to separate out the influence of each of these forces because more than one factor may be operating at the same time. Suppose that a person is receiving signals and messages that "thin is good," leading to disorders such as anorexia or bulimia. Those messages might be coming from his or her parents, siblings, other family members, friends, or the mass media, or, more likely, some combination of these forces. Yet research has been able to sort out the types of influence that each of these factors may have on an individual.

Family forces, to the extent they exist, may be strong simply because of the close, long-standing, and meaningful relationship that typically exists among families. On occasion a parent my feel that his or her child is "too fat" and transmits that feeling, either intentionally or accidentally, to the child. Or, in a similar mechanism, a child or adolescent may already be predisposed to wanting to lose weight, and parental attitudes may only support or encourage (again, intentionally or not) those feelings. A rich body of research is now available on parental characteristics that may explain a predisposition to a child's development of eating disorders. These factors tend to fall into about five general categories:

- A tendency for parents to being overprotective or overinvolved of a child
- A parent's desire for high achievement, approaching levels of perfection, in a child

- A general concern over a child's physical appearance, such as his or her seeming to be "too fat," in a parent's view

- Parental concern about a child's ability to function success-fully in a social setting that may result in the child's rejection by peers or adult figures

- An inability or unwillingness by parents to recognize or be open to a discussion of emotional issues in a child's life that may lead to an eating disorder (among the consider-able body of research on this issue, see Lucas 2009; Pike and Rodin 1991; Strober and Humphrey 1987; Tafà et al. 2017; Woodside et al. 2002)

One of the most interesting subsidiary questions in this dis-cussion has to do with the effect that mothers with an eat-ing disorder may have on the occurrence of a similar problem in their daughters. (There is essentially no research on similar effects of a father on his offspring's risk for eating disorders.) The question is complex because mother and daughter dyads (a mother and her child) differ significantly from each other. Also, research can ask (and has asked) about a number of dif-ferent aspects of this question, such as how a mother with an eating disorder may influence her daughter with regard to at-titudes about body image, self-confidence, assertiveness, and other mental and emotional factors. At this point, the answer to this question is that daughters of women with eating disor-ders are at greater risk for themselves developing such a condi-tion, although that simplistic generalization must be qualified by a number of factors of the type mentioned earlier (Cooley et al. 2008; Patel et al. 2002; Stitt 2012). The one bit of data that appears in a number of commentaries on mother–daughter eating disorder relationships is that the daughter of a woman with anorexia is 11 times as likely to develop that condition, and a daughter of a bulimic woman is 6 times more likely than are daughters of women without an eating disorder. (This data point has, however, also and often been used to argue for a genetic factor in the development of eating disorders, about which more will be discussed later in this chapter. Also see Fielder-Jenks 2017; Strober et al. 2000.)

In addition to the extensive research on the role of parental attitudes and actions in the development of eating disorders, a number of personal stories can be found on the Internet. As an example, a contributor to the *Psychology Today* analysis of eating disorders has written:

> When I first began therapy for my eating disorder over ten years ago, the relationship between my family and my eating disorder was obvious. My family was obviously dysfunctional—otherwise, why would I have an eating disorder. The evidence was everywhere. My mother was stressed and hovering, asking me if and when and what I had last eaten. My dad was distant and unemotional. I was angry and defiant.
>
> Looking back, the signs seemed even clearer. I didn't feel I could express my real emotions. My parents didn't want me to grow up. I didn't have a voice, and so I used my body to express myself. As my illness progressed, so did the family discord. Phone calls deteriorated into slanging matches. Home life became almost unbearably stressful. (Arnold 2011)

Another powerful force that influences a person's behavior is peer pressure. *Peer pressure* is the force that a person's friends exert on him or her to recognize and follow certain standards established by that group of friends. For example, the trend for a group of eighth graders to wear a certain brand of sneakers is likely to cause everyone in the group to buy that type of product. Researchers have found that peer pressure can be, and often is, a strong force in the development of eating disorders. That force arises when members of a peer group hold to and speak favorably about certain types of body shapes and sizes. If, for example, the members of the group make derogatory comments about someone's being "too fat," a message is sent to everyone in that group that thinness is an ideal to strive for. And that message can lead, in some cases, to members of that group falling into anorexic or bulimic patterns.

A number of studies have now found that friends' opinions and comments about one's weight and physical appearance are often important factors in the development of an eating disorder (see, e.g., Forney, Holland, and Keel 2012; Helfert and Warschburger 2013; Stice, Maxfield, and Wells 2003).

A recent study has suggested that peer pressure may be among the strongest of all forces leading to an eating disorder. In that study, researchers compared the relative effects of social media, television, and peer pressure in the development of eating disorders. They found that neither of the first two factors had a significant effect in leading to an eating disorder, while the last factor did. They concluded that "only peer competition, not television or social media use, predicted negative outcomes [in regard to eating disorders]" (Ferguson et al. 2014).

Studies of peer pressure among adults are much less common than for children and adolescents. The studies that have been done generally confirm the role of peer pressure in women and, to a lesser degree, men in the development of an eating disorder (Costa-Font and Jofre-Bonet 2013). In some populations, however, the effect is especially significant. The gay male community is such a population. A number of studies have been conducted on the occurrence of eating disorders in the community, as well as the factors responsible for its occurrence. Prevalence studies have found that eating disorders among gay men are about three times as common as in comparable groups of nongay men. Among the most common explanations for this phenomenon has been the impact on gay men of attitudes toward body image expressed by friends, sexual partners, and other peers (Dottermusch 2015; Feldman and Meyer 2007; Russell and Keel 2002).

Some of the strong forces leading to an eating disorder in childhood, adolescence, and adulthood are the career or recreational choices a person makes in her or his life. Examples of such choices include a commitment to ballet and modeling, where a slender body is most commonly encouraged and admired, and sports such as swimming and diving, figure skating, gymnastics, long-distance running, weight lifting, and wrestling, where either an attractive or especially muscular body is important. One of the most studied examples of this phenomenon is a condition known as *female athlete triad*. The condition was first described in 1992 by the Women's Task Force of the American College of Sports Medicine (Yeager et al. 1993). That action was taken because clinical studies had shown that women who take part in certain types of sports have a tendency to develop a set of three adverse medical conditions: (1) an eating disorder that results in a loss of essential nutrients in the body, which, in turn, results in (2) a dysfunction of the menstrual cycle, which, in turn, causes (3) osteoporosis, a loss of bone mass and the formation of fragile bones.

A recent update of information available on this condition notes that the complete set of three symptoms occurs quite rarely, ranging from 0 to 16 percent in populations that have been studied. But the presence of one or two of the components of the condition is much more common and can reach a prevalence of 50–60 percent in sports where a lean body is encouraged (Barrack, Ackerman, and Gibbs 2013). In the two decades since female athlete triad was first discussed, some long-term effects of the condition have been identified. These conditions include most of the same physical and emotional issues associated with eating disorders such as anorexia and bulimia themselves. In addition, a number of cardiovascular, endocrine, reproductive, skeletal, gastrointestinal, renal, and central nervous system disorders have been correlated with the triad. The triad has also been identified as the cause of anorexia in women at a rate six times as high as in female nonathletes. The triad condition has also been recognized as a contribution factor to the appearance of suicide ideation in more than

5 percent of athletes and former athletes (Nattiv et al. 2010; Thein-Nissenbaum 2013).

Eating patterns among males in certain sports, such as weight lifting and bodybuilding, show an interestingly different pattern from the one described here for women. In this case, the motivating force for males is a desire to increase body mass rather than to lose weight. This pattern was previously known as *reverse anorexia* and is now more commonly called *muscular dysmorphia*, or a dissatisfaction with the size and strength of one's muscles. Although different in many ways from weight-loss conditions such as anorexia and bulimia, muscular dysmorphia has now been proposed by some experts in the field as a category of eating disorders under the *Diagnostic and Statistical Manual of Mental Disorders* (see, e.g., Lentillon-Kaestner 2015).

Yet another factor that has been implicated in the development of eating disorders is abuse during a person's childhood. A large number of studies over the past two decades or more have asked whether emotional abuse, physical neglect, sexual abuse, or some other maltreatment during a person's early years is correlated with the development of an eating disorder later in her or his life. These studies have produced a mixed bag of results with ambiguous findings. In some cases, the connection between adverse events in a person's life can clearly be correlated with occurrence of an eating disorder later in one's life. One study of 73 Korean patients with eating disorders, for example, found a strong correlation between childhood emotional abuse, physical neglect, and sexual abuse (Kong and Bernstein 2009).

Other studies, however, have shown no correlation for any type of childhood abuse and eating disorders, a modest level of correlation, or a correlation between one or more types of eating disorders but not all eating disorders. An early (1993) review of such studies found the rate of eating disorders among those who had experienced abuse during their childhood was no different from those without eating disorders. The authors of this review pointed out, however, that so many methodological problems were present in these studies, however, that no clear-cut result could be drawn from them (Connors and Morse 1993).

As these problems were solved in later research, results were still not very clear. Some studies showed that one type of abuse, such as emotional abuse, sexual abuse, or physical abuse, was correlated with the development of eating disorders but not other forms of abuse (Fischer, Stojek, and Hartzell 2010). Still other studies found that some form of childhood abuse predisposed a person toward one type of eating disorder (e.g., anorexia or bulimia) but not other types (Sanci et al. 2008). A recent assessment of research in this field acknowledges this complex history of research on the question, along with the patterns of which we can be relatively confident and those that are still in a state of uncertainty. The authors of that review drew three conclusions from their research. They found that (1) there "was a consistent and positive association between CSA [child sexual abuse] and both BN [bulimia nervosa] and BED [binge eating disorder]"; (2) "CPA [child physical abuse] was associated with any ED [eating disorder]"; and (3) "although there were only few studies exploring CEA [child emotional abuse], a positive association of this form of abuse with both BN and BED was found" (Caslini et al. 2016).

Some authorities have also pointed to the occurrence of some significant traumatic event in a person's childhood, adolescence, or adulthood as a precipitating factor in the development of an eating disorder. Some examples of such events might be leaving one's home to attend college, parents' divorce, discovery of a major health problem, moving house, or death of a loved one. One recent review of this theme identified six events that might be associated with the development of an eating disorder. They were the occurrence and inadequate management of (1) a change of schools; (2) death of a family member; (3) changes in an important relationship; (4) change in one's place of lodging or job; (5) a significant illness that may or may not involve hospitalization; and (6) physical or emotional abuse, sexual assault, or incest (Berge et al. 2012).

A subset of this issue of special attention recently has been the effect of post-traumatic stress disorder (PTSD) on the occurrence of eating disorders. PTSD is a condition that is triggered by a person's exposure to some frightening of upsetting event, such long-term exposure to very troubling battlefield events or diagnosis of a life-threatening disease. One reason for the recent interest in PTSD and eating disorders is the effects that are being observed in military personnel who have been assigned to and returned from battle areas in Afghanistan, Iraq, Kuwait, Syria, and other locations where conflict has now been in progress for the better part of two decades. It should be noted, however, that PTSD is not exclusively a problem related to military personnel, but that can occur commonly in everyday life as a consequence of traumatic events of the types listed earlier. In fact, the great majority of research that has been conducted on the relationship of PTSD and eating disorders has involved nonmilitary men and women.

One of the most complete, if somewhat dated, surveys on this issue is an article published in 2007 by Dr. Timothy D. Brewerton at the Medical University of South Carolina. Brewerton summarized the information then known with some confidence about PTSD and eating disorders, listing 10 specific correlations:

- Childhood sexual abuse is a nonspecific factor in the development of eating disorders.
- Other forms of abuse during childhood are also a contributing factor to the development of eating disorders.
- Trauma is more commonly associated with the development of bulimia than with other types of eating disorders.
- The connection between trauma and eating disorders applies to children and adolescents as well as to adults.

- The connection between trauma and eating disorders, although less well studied, applies to men and boys as well as to women and girls.
- Eating disorders are correlated with various types of traumatic events.
- The severity of an eating disorder is not determined by the type or severity of the trauma from which it sprung.
- Trauma is correlated not only with eating disorders but also with a variety of comorbidities associated with the condition.
- Events that do not arise to a full definition of trauma or PTSD may still contribute to the development of bulimia and bulimic symptoms.
- Treatment of an eating disorder requires that the complete nature of the originating trauma or PTSD be fully explored and resolved (Brewerton 2007).

Research focusing especially on PTSD and eating disorders among current and past military personnel has been relatively sparse. That which has been conducted suggests that most of the patterns found in the general population also occur among military personnel and veterans. Some significant differences exist, however. Three factors associated with the unique character of the military experience are the effects of both combat and noncombat events, the stresses associated with strict weight and physical fitness requirements, and heightened risk of sexual trauma, an issue especially, but not exclusively, of concern to female military and veterans (Bartlett and Mitchell 2015; Litwack et al. 2014; Mitchell et al. 2012).

Possibly the most discussed environmental factor associated with eating disorders is the influence of the mass media. The term *mass media* refers to all of the forms of entertainment and information that are generally available to the general public through newspapers and magazines, radio and television, and the Internet. One feature of the mass media is that they tend, intentionally or not, to create certain standards as to how people think about certain issues. One's personal appearance is one such issue. The public is bombarded today with pictures and verbal descriptions of celebrities, such as motion picture stars, musical performers, professional athletes, models, and other "important" figures in the news. Females within this universe of personalities are often pictured as slender and lithesome, rarely, if ever, as overweight or obese. This type of body image, then, has become the ideal against which girls and women compare themselves and which they may strive to achieve in their own lives. For males, the ideal body image is quite different, with an emphasis on a muscular build to which boys and men aspire. In either case, changes in one's eating habits—sometimes dramatic changes—may seem to be necessary for an individual to achieve these objectives.

The problem with the research conducted thus far on this issue is that it has produced no clear-cut answer to the question as to whether the media are a cause of eating disorders. A variety of studies have shown that *some* types of media have *certain* kinds of effects on *some* individuals under *certain* circumstances but not others. In one of the most extensive and thorough studies of the research on this topic, the authors reported a very ambiguous, mixed finding, namely that "engagement with mass media is probably best considered a variable risk factor that might well be later shown to be a causal risk factor" (Levine and Murnen 2009, 9). A second meta-analysis of studies on the topic produced similar results. Researchers in this case concluded that "media exposure of the ideal physique results in small changes in eating disorder symptoms, particularly with participants at high risk for developing an eating disorder" (Hausenblas et al. 2012).

Biological Factors

For most of modern history, scholars have acted on the assumption that eating disorders are caused by one of two factors—the personal choices a person makes about his or her eating habits or forces in the surrounding world that may influence those choices—or some combination of the two. Yet, over recent decades, another explanation for the source of eating disorders has caught the attention of researchers: biological factors. That is, an argument can be made that a person develops anorexia, bulimia, or some other eating disorders not entirely or exclusively because of the personal decision one makes or environmental factors but because of the biological and chemical processes that take place in that person's body that predispose him or her to development of an eating disorder. This variety of etiological factors is a manifestation of the classic debate over *nature versus nurture*. That is, do people behave the way they do because of bodily structure and function over which they have little or no control (nature) or because of social, cultural, and other external factors that act on a person to produce certain behaviors (nurture)?

That debate has gone on over hundreds of years, resulting in a general consensus that human behavior generally reflects both forces working on a person. Some behaviors, however, are more likely the result of biological factors (nature) and others the consequence of external forces (nurture). It is important in understanding human behaviors such as eating anomalies, however, to ferret out the specific biological and environmental forces at work and the relative impact of those forces.

Genetic Factors

An interest in biological factors in the production of eating disorders is easy to understand. Any number of studies have discovered that eating disorders tend to "run in a family." As noted earlier, for example, a girl whose mother is anorexic stands about 11 times the risk of becoming anorexic also than does a girl whose mother is not anorexic. Data of this kind cannot help but cause a researcher to wonder the source of that hereditary connection. It could be, of course (and also as noted earlier), that simply being part of a family that contains an anorexic mother can increase the risk that a daughter will develop the same condition: an environmental cause. But there is now evidence that some portion of that correlation exists because of hereditary factors that are passed down from generation to generation, usually mother to daughter.

It is for this reason, then, that a search for genetic factors that may be responsible for the development of eating disorders has become ever more popular in recent years. That research has been increasingly productive because of the rapid improvement in methods for studying DNA, the chemical material of which genes are composed. Today, the vast majority of research on the genetic causes of eating disorders could never have been carried out even a few decades ago, without these developments. Today it is possible to trace even the smallest variation in the chemical structure of a gene from its "normal" appearance, a change that might result in some body "abnormality."

Such research is, however, profoundly challenging for a number of reasons. In the first place, most scholars believe that only very small changes (mutations) in a gene may be involved in the development of an eating disorder. It may involve a process somewhat like searching for a "needle in a haystack" to find these minuscule gene modifications. Also, most researchers believe that more than one—probably a good many—gene mutations are involved in eating disorders. The way in which those genes interact with each other to produce the final result is another serious challenge. Another factor increasing the complexity of this research is the interaction that takes place between genetic changes and the environment. Genes do not necessarily *cause* a disorder; they may also simply *predispose* a person to that disorder. In such a case, the expression of the gene(s) may depend on environmental forces that encourage or discourage actual physical and biological events.

Fortunately, developments in DNA technology have now teased out the genetic basis for a number of developmental disabilities, disorders whose origin was largely unknown a few decades ago but for which specific genes have now been found. Disorders for which genetic causes have now been identified include anxiety disorder, autism, attention deficit hyperactivity disorder, major depression, bipolar disorder, and addiction (Vorstman and Ophoff 2013). Comparable research on eating disorders has been slow, however. Some reviews in the mid- to late 2000s have described the efforts made to that point and the findings of that research (Poyastro Pinheiro, Root, and Bulik 2009).

By the early 2010s, however, some early successes were being reported. For example, one team of researchers reported that they had conducted a broad study of the DNA of 1,003 patients with anorexia compared to a control group of 3,733 pediatric subjects. They found no correlation that specifically correlate any part of a genome with the eating disorder but found "suggestive evidence" that certain segments of DNA might be associated with the disorder. They concluded that their results "point to intriguing genes that await further validation in independent cohorts for confirmatory roles in AN [anorexia nervosa]" (Wang et al. 2010, 949).

Somewhat later, another group of researchers reported on their research on two "large families" in which anorexia appeared to be transmitted from generation to generation. They found mutations in two genes that appeared to be related to the development of anorexia. One gene, the estrogen-related receptor α (*ESRRA*) gene, has been implicated in control of the metabolic process in humans. The other gene, the histone deacetylase 4 (*HDAC4*) gene, has been found to affect a variety of steps involved in a person's physical development (Cui et al. 2013). Similar results were reported a year later when a large (47 members) research team obtained evidence for a correlation between the epoxide hydrolase 2 (*EPHX2*) gene. This gene functions in the synthesis of cholesterol in the human body and has been associated with the determination of a person's BMI (Scott-Van Zeeland et al. 2014).

The most ambitious research study currently under way is the Anorexia Nervosa Genetics Initiative (ANGI) conducted at the University of North Carolina under the auspices of the Klarman Family Foundation. The study was announced in May 2013 and has been described as "the largest and most rigorous genetic investigation of eating disorders ever conducted" (ANGI—Anorexia Nervosa Genetics Initiative 2017). Researchers from Australia, Denmark, Sweden, and the United States plan to collect data and blood samples from more than 8,000 individuals worldwide in an attempt to find genetic anomalies that are associated with anorexia nervosa. In its spring 2015 halfway update, researchers announced that they had already collected 7,000 blood samples and had raised their goal to 13,000 such samples in the remaining two years of the project (Anorexia Nervosa Genetics Initiative: Spring Update 2015; for more details, see Arnold 2013).

Other Biological Factors

Various hypotheses about other biological causes of eating disorders have been proposed. These hypotheses focus on bodily characteristics and changes that are more easily studied and measured than are the genetic factors discussed thus far. One common area of research, for example, is focused on hormonal differences that may exist between individuals with an eating disorder and others who do not have the condition. Hormones are chemical "messengers" that control many essential functions of the human body. One well-known hormone is insulin, which controls the amount of glucose ("sugar") in a person's body. Hormones are produced in a variety of glands and travel to all parts of the body to make possible the functions needed to keep a person alive and healthy. The major hormone-producing glands in the human body are the pituitary, thyroid, parathyroid, and adrenal glands, along with the pancreas, ovaries, and testes. The set of glands and hormones in the human body are known as the *endocrine system*. Because hormones often control, and are controlled by, parts of the nervous system, the endocrine system is also commonly known as the *neuroendocrine system*.

A good deal of research has been devoted to a study of a region of the brain known as the hypothalamic–pituitary–adrenal axis, which controls a number of essential bodily functions in humans. Although the interactions of these three glands are very complex, a common line of action involves the stimulation of the hypothalamus by a chemical agent or physical force, causing the release of one or more hormones to the pituitary gland, which, in turn, stimulates the release of one or more hormones from the pituitary gland to the adrenal glands. Finally, the adrenal glands release their own hormones that target the digestive, reproductive, and other systems. As one specific example, one region of the hypothalamus, called the *lateral hypothalamus*, produces a sensation of hunger when stimulated. It produces hormones that send a message to the brain that says "I want to eat." A second region of the hypothalamus, called the *ventromedial hypothalamus*, produces the opposite sensation—satiation—when it is stimulated. When stimulated, the ventromedial hypothalamus sends a message to the brain that says "I'm full," and a person loses interesting in eating. If either of these portions of the brain is damaged or defective, a person's eating habits are likely to be affected: an unending desire for food (trending toward binge eating disorder, bulimia, overweight, and obesity) if the ventromedial hypothalamus is involved or a lack of interest in eating (anorexia) if the lateral hypothalamus is involved (Smith and Ferguson 2008).

Research studies have also focused on the role of specific biochemical compounds in the development of eating disorders. Among the hormones for which some evidence exists of an effect on eating patterns are T4, estradiol, testosterone, insulin-like growth factor 1, growth hormone (GH), cortisol, leptin, adiponectin, ghrelin, and peptide YY (PYY; peptide tyrosine

tyrosine). In some cases, an increase in the concentration of a hormone may be associated with the development of an eating disorder, or a decrease in another hormone may have a similar effect. For example, current research suggests that a higher level of GH is associated with the occurrence of anorexia (for more details on the terminology, nature, and action of these hormones, see Warren 2011).

An example of the possible hormonal influences on appetite involves the two compounds, ghrelin and leptin. The former is an *orexigenic* hormone, one that stimulates appetite, while the latter is an *anorexigenic* hormone, one that reduces appetite. Normally there is a balance between the two hormones, found primarily in the stomach, that encourages a person to eat (ghrelin) but to stop eating when one is full (leptin), which helps maintain a normal body mass. There is now strong suggestive evidence, however, that individuals in whom one or the other hormone predominates may have a tendency toward the development of anorexia or bulimia (leptin) or binge eating or obesity (ghrelin). Such research is still in its early stages, however, and more studies are needed to clarify the precise nature of this relationship (Atalayer et al. 2013; Monteleone and Maj 2013).

Binge Eating, Overweight, and Obesity

At first glance, the eating disorders of anorexia and bulimia would seem to have very different causes than disorders such as binge eating and obesity. In the former case, the most characteristic property of the disorder is self-starvation and weight loss. The latter case, on the other hand, is characterized by weight gains. Still, researchers have pointed to a number of similarities between the two types of eating disorders. There is now evidence to suggest that many of the causes described earlier leading to anorexic disorders may also influence a person to gain weight rather than lose it. Such factors include psychological factors, such as anxiety, depression, PTSD, OCD, panic disorders, and phobias; environmental factors, such as sexual or physical abuse or family influences; and biological factors, such as the presence of certain genetic traits or biological reactions, such as those between ghrelin and leptin. Indeed, the list of factors responsible for binge eating disorder tends to closely match the list for anorexic conditions (Binge Eating Disorder 2017; Day, Ternouth, and Collier 2009; Eating Disorders and Obesity: How Are They Related? n.d.).

The increasing incidence of obesity in the United States and other parts of the world has motivated an aggressive program of research to discover the causes of overweight that go beyond those mentioned in the previous paragraph. That research has produced a large and complex set of factors that may contribute significantly or in modest ways to the development of obesity. At this point, which of these factors are of greatest importance and how those factors may interact with each is the subject of an intensive debate among obesity researchers (for one of the best-available articles on this issue, see McAllister et al. 2009). On the simplest possible level, there is a general agreement that obesity occurs when the balance between diet and exercise is disrupted. That is, a healthy human needs to take in a certain number of calories each day to maintain body systems and stay healthy. Normal bodily processes such as walking, running, working, and thinking then require the expenditure of a certain number of those calories. If caloric intake is roughly equal to caloric expenditures, one neither gains nor loses weight, the most desirable condition. If one takes in an excess of calories (eats too much) or expends too future calories (does not exercise the body to a desirable extent), one tends to gain weight. And the greater the excess of calories taken in over calories expended, the more weight one gains. This basic relationship leads to the most common advice given to avoid overweight and obesity: eat less and/or exercise more.

This fundamental relationship does not really answer the question as to *why* a person adopts an unbalanced caloric program. What *causes* a person to eat more and exercise less than he or she should? A number of answers have been suggested for that question. Experts do not agree on the extent, if any, to which each of the following factors contributes to a person's tendency toward obesity, but all have been proposed at one time or another by one research team or another. (Relevant factors such as genetic, biological, familial, peer pressure, and emotional mentioned earlier are not repeated here.)

- Certain diseases, especially those that are genetic in origin and/or may involve the endocrine system, may increase a person's risk for overweight and obesity. Those diseases include Alström syndrome, Bardet-Biedl syndrome, Cohen syndrome, Cushing's syndrome, hypothyroidism, insulin resistance, polycystic ovary syndrome, and Prader-Willi syndrome (Lee and Mattson 2014; Weaver 2008).

- Certain medications may also be a factor in the development of obesity, such as certain anticonvulsants, antidepressants, antihistamines, and antipsychotics; some high blood pressure drugs; most corticosteroids; insulin; some oral contraceptives; and members of the sulfonylurea and thiazolidinedione families (Keith et al. 2006; McAllister et al. 2009).

- A poor choice of eating patterns, which could mean selecting portion sizes larger than necessary for good health; choosing foods high in calories, saturated fats, high-fructose corn syrup, or other less nutritious ingredients; eating out frequently; eating for reasons other than the maintenance of good health, such as choosing "comfort foods" to make one feel better under emotional stress; consuming too many sugary drinks, such as colas; selecting foods from vending machines, which tend to be less nutritious than foods from other sources; *not* including especially important foods, such as fruits and vegetables, in one's diet; and consumption of alcoholic drinks (Food and Diet 2017).

- Sleep deprivation has also been implicated in the development of obesity. A number of studies now suggest that individuals who become sleep deprived, for whatever reason, have an increased tendency to gain weight. A number of explanations for this fact have been suggested, such as the hormonal changes that may accompany sleep deprivation, emotional problems that may be the cause of sleep problem, and the simple fact that people who sleep less may have a greater opportunity to eat more often (Obesity and Sleep 2017; Patel and Hu 2008).

- The food environment is now thought to be a powerful factor in the growth in obesity rates in the United States and other developed countries. As used here, the term *food environment* refers to all of the ways in which foods are made available to the general public. It includes advertising by food producers and distributors, the composition of food available to the public, portion sizes used in commercial food establishments and other food outlets, and the nutritional value of commercially available food. There is little disagreement about the fact that an individual today has a much wider choice of foods than did our even recent ancestors, most of whom relied on foods produced around their homes or in nearby farms. Today, people have a choice of foods produced in all parts of the world, often in a highly processed form with reduced nutritional value. These processed foods tend to be high in simple carbohydrates, saturated fats, food additives, and other components with little or no nutritional value. As a consequence, the public is more likely to consume foods that are high in calories and low in nutritional value.

  - Food companies also tend to promote these products aggressively in newspapers and magazines, on radio and television, in motion pictures, and on social media. These advertisements have been implicated in the increase in weight problems recently recorded among underserved and lower-class populations and especially among children.

  - The manner in which foods are presented commercially can also be a factor in the development of obesity. Fast-food restaurants and other food outlets have tended to increase the portion size of their products in recent decades, increasing the number of calories consumed by an individual who eats at such locations (Jolly 2011; for an excellent introduction to the problems of obesity in general, see Stern and Kazaks 2015).

- In addition to these relatively well-known and widely discussed causes of obesity, a number of less obvious factors have been hypothesized and studied. Many of these factors are ones that the average person might not imagine as being a cause of obesity; yet research suggests that most are worthy of study as possible risk factors for obesity. For example, one group of authors has suggested that humans who are placed in an environment where the temperature is significantly greater than or less than that needed for maintenance of good health are at reduced risk for weight gain. Thus, the greater availability of air-conditioning and central heat allows people to live in their "comfort zone," which requires fewer calories to body maintenance. These calories are then turned into weight gain (McAllister et al. 2009). The authors conclude their long study of obesity factors by suggesting that "multiple plausible causes of obesity [such as ambient temperature] exist outside of the big two [food marketing practices and reduction in physical activity] and that as of yet these alternatives have had little if any influence on mainstream discussions of clinical and public health approaches to obesity. This is unfortunate because some of these putative causes could lead directly to practical intervention and prevention approaches" (McAllister et al. 2009).

Prevention and Treatment of Eating Disorders

Prevention

As with any other disease or disorder, finding ways of preventing the condition rather than spending resources on treating it is the preferable approach to dealing with the condition.

Prevention programs for eating disorders are generally classified into one of three categories: universal, selective, and indicated (or targeted), also known as primary, secondary, and tertiary. (This system was first proposed in 1983 by Robert S. Gordon. See Gordon 1983. Some authorities use a somewhat different scheme for categorizing types of prevention programs.) Universal programs are aimed at groups of individuals, whether they are specifically at risk for an eating disorder or not. Such programs might be carried out at the national, state, regional, or local levels. They might also be directed at specialized groups, such as students at schools or colleges. The objective of these programs is to provide a wide range of individuals with information about the causes and nature of eating disorders. The assumption is that this information will reduce the likelihood that members of the target group will engage in eating disorder behaviors (Kroon Van Diest and Perez 2012; Wilksch 2014). In practice, the vast majority of universal prevention programs are designed for school groups ranging from early primary to late high school levels, plus college and university populations. (For examples of such programs, with descriptions of their approaches and evaluations of their success, see Stice and Shaw 2004, 210–212, table 1.)

Selective programs are designed for populations known to be at risk for the development of eating disorders. Examples of such populations are girls and women, athletes, and dancers. Again, the primary objective of such programs is to make sure that individuals are well informed about the risks posed by eating disorders and, armed with that information, willing to take whatever actions are necessary to avoid developing an eating disorder. Some common objectives of selective programs are as follows:

- Helping an individual recognize the costs of adopting the cultural body ideal of "thin" (for girls) or "muscular and lean" (for boys)
- Encouraging the acceptance of balanced attitudes on body image, eating, and weight

- Recognizing that body shape and weight are not productive standards for defining personal success, happiness, and self-worth
- Providing education on the physical and psychological risks of eating disorders
- Outlining the basic principles of a program of balanced nutrition and physical activity (Adapted from Awareness, Prevention, and Early Intervention 2016)

Indicated prevention programs are designed for individuals who exhibit signs and symptoms of a specific eating disorder but are not yet at a stage where they can be categorized as anorexic or bulimic. As an example, a woman may begin to realize that she has become obsessed by her body shape and size and understands that this may be the first step in developing a full-blown eating disorder. If that individual makes known her pre-disorder concerns, she is a candidate for an indicated prevention program. Such programs attempt to interrupt the progress of the individual from simply be "at risk" to developing a full-blown eating disorder.

All prevention programs use one or more techniques for dealing with problems associated with eating disorders. One of the most popular is called cognitive dissonance, an approach in which counselors attempt to provide an individual with an image or understanding of an issue that is in conflict with one already held by the individual. For example, cognitive dissonance intervention for a person who has adopted the ideal body image presented in some media may include specific examples of successful individuals whose body does not conform to that ideal. Another approach, often called *media literacy*, aims to help individuals develop a better understanding of how the media works and the messages it may attempt to purvey. A third approach is called *motivational interviewing*. In this method, a counselor works with an individual to understand the differences between one's current beliefs and thoughts about eating disorders to a new and more healthful understanding of those issues. (For examples of the approaches to prevention programs described here, see For Schools; In the Community; Sports & Fitness Industry 2017.)

Probably the key question associated with prevention programs is, "Do they work?" If so, which programs in which formats appear to be most successful? This question has been studied on a number of occasions, with sometimes contradictory and confusing results. Research on the topic has been complicated by the complexity of the question itself. Studies have differed in the number of participants involved, the method used in the study, the variables being investigated, the length of time the program was in operation, definitions used as to the "success" of the program, and other variables. Currently, the consensus of these studies appears to be that, yes, prevention programs *can* be successful, at least to some extent, provided that certain criteria are met. As one pair of researchers has observed,

> Overall, empirical evidence supports the effectiveness of several eating disorder prevention programs, with most programs decreasing current and future eating disorder symptoms and associated risk factors. More importantly, some of these effects have been sustained for extended periods of time. (Kroon Van Diest and Perez 2012, 309)

Another meta-analysis, on the other hand, takes note of a trend observed in a number of studies, namely that individuals who have taken part in a prevention program do show improvements in knowledge about eating disorder issues. However, they tend not to show much change in the behaviors they exhibit in that regard. That is, such participants know more about eating disorders but are not much less inclined to put that knowledge into practice (Langmesser and Verscheure 2009).

Finally, a meta-analysis of meta-analyses (a review of meta-analysis studies) on the efficacy of eating disorder prevention programs summarized a number of factors that appear to be most strongly associated with successful programs. The results of this study are probably in line with those that might be expected from such studies. Specifically, they are as follows:

- Selective programs tend to be more effective than universal programs, probably because participants in the former are more motivated to make changes than are those in the latter. A few studies have shown different results, with universal programs being superior to or at least equal in effectiveness to selective programs.

- Programs involving adolescents tend to be more successful than those designed for adults. The reason may be that eating disorders arise most commonly during teen years than at older ages, so interventions during this period are likely to have a greater probability of success.

- The type of program personnel appears to be a factor in the likelihood of success of a program. Individuals who have been especially trained to take part in such programs seem to produce better results than are those without special training, such as teachers, nurses, and school counselors.

- Content of a program is also a mediating factor in that interactional programs, in which individuals take part in the educational process, are more effective than those in which information is provided by teaching (classical didactic) methods (all items from Shaw, Stice, and Becker 2009; also see Cororve Fingeret et al. 2006; Le et al. 2017; Levine 2015).

A very important final conclusion about research on the effectiveness of prevention programs, however, is that diverse results have been reported in all of these areas, and some questions still remain about the best way to help the general population and those at risk for eating disorders to deal with this issue.

One of the issues that has caused some concern among clinicians is the possibility of producing iatrogenic effects during prevention programs. An *iatrogenic effect* is an unexpected, inadvertent, and usually undesirable change as the result of some medical treatment. In the case of eating disorders, for example, there have been reports of an individual's developing anorexia or bulimia *as a consequence* of a prevention or treatment program (see, e.g., Raven 2016). Some modest evidence exists or suggests that such effects may occur among patients in prevention or treatment programs (Garner 1985; Strober 2004; Tetyana 2012). Because of these concerns and anecdotal reports of iatrogenic effects, a number of studies of prevention programs have included questions about the frequency with which such effects occur. Those studies appear to show that such effects as so rare as to of modest concern among researchers, and iatrogenic effects are generally not considered to be a drawback in well-designed and well-executed prevention programs (see, e.g., Cororve Fingeret et al. 2006; Langmesser and Verscheure 2009; Stice and Shaw 2004).

Treatment

Treatment of eating disorders differs substantially from person to person depending on a number of factors, including the cost of treatment, type of specialization of counselors, insurance coverage, and distance from one's home. (For an excellent review of these factors, see Selecting a Treatment Center for Your Loved One 2017.) Probably the most important of these factors is the nature and severity of a person's eating disorder. As with other types of physical diseases and mental disorders, treatment programs are available for everyone from the person who is showing no signs or symptoms of an eating disorder (but may be at risk for the problem) to someone who is so ill that his or her life is at risk. A variety of facilities are available for this range of problems:

• Outpatient treatment: Designed for individuals with the lowest level of concern regarding eating disorders. A person meets with a dietician, nutritionist, psychologist, psychiatrist, or other specialist in the field for a few hours a few days each week.

- Day treatment: A person who has somewhat more serious issues than an outpatient. The individual usually spends a typical "workday," from 8:00 A.M. to 5:00 P.M., five days a week, at a specialized center for treatment. The patient then returns home in the evening and stays at home on weekends.

- Residential inpatient treatment: An individual has been diagnosed with a full-blown eating disorder or has reached a stage very close to that condition. The person checks into a specialized facility whose sole purpose it is to treat eating disorder patients. The facility has developed a complete program of education, nutritional services, counseling, and other services to deal with one or more types of eating disorder. (An extensive list of treatment facilities in the United States can be found at Eating Disorder Treatment Center 2017.)

- Hospitals: Hospital treatment is required when an individual has become physically or mentally unstable and requires round-the-clock intensive medical and/or psychiatric care. Individuals provided with this level of care may have reached a life-threatening status.

(For a detailed list of criteria leading to the choice of one or another type of treatment facility, see Treatment Settings and Levels of Care 2017.)

The components of a treatment program for an eating disorder are roughly comparable. Patients are encouraged to identify and understand the factors that have led to their condition and then to develop mechanisms for reducing the impact of those factors. A typical treatment program might include, for example, individual counseling with a psychologist, nutritionist, social worker, or other specialist in the field; family counseling sessions; therapy groups that use a variety of techniques including cognitive behavioral therapy, interpersonal therapy, dialectical behavioral therapy, art therapy, or animal therapy; nutritional counseling; and medication management. Inpatient programs rely on most of these treatment modalities, with more time being spent, as permitted by the full-time presence of an individual in the program. In some cases, a greater choice of therapies may also be available, such as specialized groups focusing on psychoeducation, body image, family dynamics, art therapy, motivation for change, movement therapy, self-esteem, creative visualization of meals, healthy sports management, nutrition education, food preparation, horticulture, parenting, occupational therapy, relapse prevention, PTSD, substance abuse, and stress management (Inpatient Program 2017; also see Understanding Anorexia Treatment: What to Expect during the First Week in Residential Treatment 2015).

The most aggressive form of treatment for eating disorders involves full-time hospitalization. This approach is indicated when a person's physical and/or medical condition has deteriorated to a degree that intensive professional treatment may be needed just to keep the patient alive and to deal with the cardiovascular, gastrointestinal, endocrine, metabolic, hematologic, neurologic, ophthalmic, and pulmonary issues that may be associated with advanced cases of anorexia, bulimia, and other eating disorders. While in the hospital, a patient will probably also be provided with many of the same services and therapies available for outpatient and inpatient individuals, although perhaps at a most intensive level.

An additional type of treatment program may be offered to individuals who have completed a hospital stay and are ready to return to a more normal life. This partial hospitalization treatment requires that a person participate in an intensive 12-hour-a-day, 7-days-a-week program of therapy and counseling similar to that available in inpatient programs but, again, with a more aggressive agenda.

A substantial body of research has been devoted to an analysis of the efficacy of various types of treatment programs. That research is especially difficult because of the variety of eating disorders involved, the type of patients who take part in treatment, the specific varieties of treatment programs, and other factors. One review of such studies commented on the consequences of this complex mix of factors. It noted that "although potentially useful in guiding treatment selection, consistent predictors of treatment outcome have not been identified in eating disorders." The same review highlighted one very specific successful treatment: the use of cognitive behavioral therapy for the treatment of bulimia and binge eating disorder. Findings for other therapies, however, were mixed and ambiguous. These results suggested that two other factors also be taken into consideration in the choice of a treatment program: clinical expertise and certain patient characteristics. Finally, as with many such studies, the authors concluded that "future investigations are critical, particularly to determine more efficacious eating disorder treatments" (Peterson et al. 2016).

Conclusion

Eating disorder issues present complex challenges for researchers, clinicians, patients, and their families and friends. The variety of possible disorders, from self-starvation to overeating phenomena, and the wide range of possible factors responsible for such conditions make diagnosis, prevention, and treatment difficult problems for all who are involved. A great deal has been learned about eating disorders over the past half century, but, as most experts in the field now accept, much more research needs to be done and better methods for implementing current research findings must be found.

References

Adkins, Havilah. 2017. "Anorexia Nervosa and Bone Densitometry." *Radiologic Technology*. 88(4): 401–418. https://media.asrt.org/pdf/drpubs/RADT_Vol88_No4_ANBD_DR.pdf. Accessed on May 9, 2017.

Allen, Karina L., et al. 2014. "Risk Factors for Binge Eating and Purging Eating Disorders: Differences Based on Age of Onset." *International Journal of Eating Disorders*. 47(7): 802–812.

"ANGI—Anorexia Nervosa Genetics Initiative." 2017. Center of Excellence for Eating Disorders. University of North Carolina. http://www.med.unc.edu/psych/eatingdisorders/ our-research/angi/angi-anorexia-nervosa-genetics-initiative. Accessed on May 28, 2017.

"Anorexia Nervosa." 2015. The Center for Eating Disorders. https://www.eatingdisorder.org/eating-disorder-information/anorexia-nervosa/. Accessed on May 6, 2017.

"Anorexia Nervosa Genetics Initiative: Spring 2015 Update." 2015. Center of Excellence for Eating Disorders. University of North Carolina. https://uncexchanges.org/2017/08/30/ anorexia-nervosa-genetics-initiative-an-update-2/. Accessed on November 27, 2018.

Arnold, Carrie. 2011. "The Real Relationship between Families and Eating Disorders." *Psychology Today*. https:// www.psychologytoday.com/blog/body-evidence/201107/ the-real-relationship-between-families-and-eating-disorders. Accessed on May 22, 2017.

Arnold, Carrie. 2013. "Finding Better Genes—The Anorexia Nervosa Genetics Initiative." ED Bites. http://edbites .com/2013/05/angi/. Accessed on May 28, 2017.

Atalayer, Deniz, et al. 2013. "Ghrelin and Eating Disorders." *Progress in Neuropsychopharmacology & Biological Psychiatry*. 40: 70–82. https://www.ncbi.nlm .nih.gov/pmc/articles/PMC3522761/. Accessed on May 30, 2017.

Attri, Navneet, et al. 2008. "Rumination Syndrome: An Emerging Case Scenario." *Southern Medical Journal*. 101(4): 432–435. http://www.medscape.com/viewarticle/573182. Accessed on May 8, 2017.

"Awareness, Prevention, and Early Intervention." 2016. National Eating Disorders Collaboration. http://www.nedc .com.au/primary-prevention. Accessed on June 3, 2017.

Bachar, Eytan, et al. 2008. "Surgery and Parental Separation as Potential Risk Factors for Abnormal Eating Attitudes— Longitudinal Study." *European Eating Disorders Review.* 16(6): 442–450. https://www.academia.edu/18057517/ Surgery_and_parental_separation_as_potential_risk_ factors_for_abnormal_eating_attitudes-longitudinal_ study?auto=download. Accessed on May 17, 2017.

Barbarich, Nicole C., Walter H. Kaye, and David Jimerson. 2003. "Neurotransmitter and Imaging Studies in Anorexia Nervosa: New Targets for Treatment." *Current Drug Target—CNS & Neurological Disorders.* 2(1): 61–72.

Barrack, Michelle T., Kathryn E. Ackerman, and Jenna C. Gibbs. 2013. "Update on the Female Athlete Triad." *Current Reviews in Musculoskeletal Medicine.* 6(2): 195–204.

Bartlett, Brooke A., and Karen S. Mitchell. 2015. "Eating Disorders in Military and Veteran Men and Women: A Systematic Review." *International Journal of Eating Disorders.* 48(8): 1057–1069.

Battiste, Nikki, and Lauren Effron. 2012. "EDNOS: Deadliest Eating Disorder Is Quietly the Most Common." ABC News. http://abcnews.go.com/Health/ednos-deadliest-eating-disorder-quietly-common/story?id=17709815. Accessed on May 14, 2017.

Bell, Leigh. 2015. "Electrolytes and Bulimia: Why Is This a Big Deal?" Eating Disorder Hope. https://www.eating disorderhope.com/information/bulimia/electrolytes-and-bulimia-why-is-this-a-big-deal. Accessed on May 12, 2017.

Bemporad, Jules R. 1997. "Cultural and Historical Aspects of Eating Disorders." *Theoretical Medicine.* 18(4): 401–420.

http://brown.uk.com/eatingdisorders/bemporad.pdf. Accessed on May 18, 2017.

Berge, Jerica M., et al. 2012. "Family Life Cycle Transitions and the Onset of Eating Disorders: A Retrospective Grounded Theory Approach." *Journal of Clinical Nursing*. 21(9–10): 1355–1363. https://www.ncbi.nlm .nih.gov/pmc/articles/PMC3207010/. Accessed on May 25, 2017.

Bhandari, Smitha. 2016. "Mental Health and Rumination Disorder." WebMD. http://www.webmd.com/mental-health/rumination-disorder#1. Accessed on May 8, 2017.

"Binge Eating Disorder." 2017. PsychGuides.com. http://www .psychguides.com/guides/binge-eating-disorder/#effects. Accessed on May 12, 2017.

Blue, Miranda. 2015. "RWW News: Pat Robertson: Eating Disorders 'Can Be Treated as a Demonic Possession.' " YouTube. https://www.youtube.com/watch?v=6oWzxhixxqQ. Accessed on May 18, 2017.

Bratman, Steven. 2017. Orthorexia. http://www.orthorexia .com/. Accessed on May 13, 2017.

Brewerton, Timothy D. 2007. "Eating Disorders, Trauma, and Comorbidity: Focus on PTSD." *Eating Disorders*. 15(4): 285–304. https://www.researchgate.net/ publication/6128514_Eating_Disorders_Trauma_and_ Comorbidity_Focus_on_PTSD. Accessed on May 26, 2017.

Brown, Carrie A. 2017. "The Physical Side Effects of Bulimia." Eating Disorder Hope. https://www.eatingdisorderhope .com/information/bulimia/the-physical-side-effects-of-buli mia. Accessed on May 12, 2017.

Buckner, Julia D., Jose Silgado, and Peter M. Lewinsohn. 2010. "Delineation of Differential Temporal Relations between Specific Eating and Anxiety Disorders." *Journal of Psychiatric Research*. 44(12): 781–787. https://www

.researchgate.net/publication/41577855_Delineation_
of_differential_temporal_relations_between_eating_and_
anxiety_disorders. Accessed on May 21, 2017.

Bühren, K., et al. 2014. "Comorbid Psychiatric Disorders in
Female Adolescents with First-Onset Anorexia Nervosa."
European Eating Disorders Review. 22(1): 39–44.

Bulik, Cynthia. 2002. "Eating Disorders in Adolescents and
Young Adults." *Child and Adolescent Psychiatric Clinics of
North America.* 11(2): 201–218.

"Bulimia Nervosa." 2017. Mayo Clinic. http://www
.mayoclinic.org/diseases-conditions/bulimia/symptoms-
causes/dxc-20179827. Accessed on May 7, 2017.

Caslini, Manuela, et al. 2016. "and Eating Disorders:
A Systematic Review and Meta-analysis." *Psychosomatic
Medicine.* 78(1): 79–90. https://www.researchgate.net/
publication/281772409_Disentangling_the_Association_
Between_Child_Abuse_and_Eating_Disorders_A_
Systematic_Review_and_Meta-Analysis. Accessed on
May 25, 2017.

Connors, Mary E., and Wayne Morse. 1993. "Sexual Abuse
and Eating Disorders: A Review." *International Journal of
Eating Disorders.* 13(1): 1–11.

Cooley, Eric, et al. 2008. "Maternal Effects on Daughters' Eating
Pathology and Body Image." *Eating Behaviors.* 9(1): 52–61.

Cororve Fingeret, Michelle, et al. 2006. "Eating Disorder
Prevention Research: A Meta-analysis." *Eating Disorders.*
14(3): 191–213. https://www.researchgate.net/
publication/6977909_Eating_Disorder_Prevention_
Research_A_Meta-Analysis. Accessed on June 4, 2017.

Costa-Font, Joan, and Mireia Jofre-Bonet. 2013. "Anorexia,
Body Image and Peer Effects: Evidence from a Sample of
European Women." *Economica.* 80(317): 44–64.

Cui, Huxing, et al. 2013. "Eating Disorder Predisposition Is
Associated with ESRRA and HDAC4 Mutations." *Journal*

of Clinical Investigations. 123(11): 4706–4713. https://www.jci.org/articles/view/71400/pdf. Accessed on May 29, 2017.

Curie, Alan. 2010. "Sport and Eating Disorders—Understanding and Managing the Risks." *Asian Journal of Sports Medicine.* 1(2): 63–68.

Daluiski, Aaron, Bita Rahbar, and Roy A. Meals. 1997. "Russell's Sign: Subtle Hand Changes in Patients with Bulimia Nervosa." *Clinical Orthopaedics and Related Research.* 343: 107–109.

Day, Jemma, Andrew Ternouth, and David A. Collier. 2009. "Eating Disorders and Obesity: Two Sides of the Same Coin?" *Epidemiologia e Psichiatria Sociale.* 18(2): 96–100.

Dell'Osso, Liliana, et al. 2016. "Historical Evolution of the Concept of Anorexia Nervosa and Relationships with Orthorexia Nervosa, Autism, and Obsessive—Compulsive Spectrum." *Neuropsychiatric Disease and Treatment.* 12: 1651–1660. https://www.ncbi.nlm.nih.gov/pmc/articles/PMC4939998/. Accessed on April 24, 2017.

Denholm, M., and J. Jankowski. 2011. "Gastroesophageal Reflux Disease and Bulimia Nervosa—A Review of the Literature." *Diseases of the Esophagus.* 24(2): 79–85.

"Diseases and Conditions: Obesity. Risk Factors." 2017. Mayo Clinic. http://www.mayoclinic.org/diseases-conditions/obesity/basics/risk-factors/con-20014834. Accessed on May 18, 2017.

Dottermusch, Megan. 2015. "Eating Disorders: The Secret Epidemic Facing Gay Men." Adios Barbie. http://www.adiosbarbie.com/2015/03/eating-disorders-the-secret-epidemic-facing-gay-men/. Accessed on May 24, 2017.

Dynesen, Anja Weirsøe, et al. 2008. "Salivary Changes and Dental Erosion in Bulimia Nervosa." *Oral Surgery, Oral Medicine, Oral Pathology, Oral Radiology and Endodontology.* 106(5): 696–707.

"Eating Disorder Treatment Centers." 2017. Eating Disorder Hope. https://www.eatingdisorderhope.com/treatment-centers. Accessed on June 5, 2017.

"Eating Disorders." 2017. National Institute of Mental Health. https://www.nimh.nih.gov/health/topics/eating-disorders/index.shtml. Accessed on May 7, 2017.

"Eating Disorders and Obesity: How Are They Related?" n.d. BodyWorks. http://www.nkfm.org/sites/default/files/documents/pages/eating_disorders_obesity.pdf. Accessed on May 31, 2017.

"Eating Disorders in LGBT Populations." 2017. National Eating Disorders Association. https://www.nationaleating disorders.org/eating-disorders-lgbt-populations. Accessed on May 17, 2017.

"Eating Disorders—The Physical and Psychological Consequences of Eating Disorders." 2017. faqs.org. http://www.faqs.org/health/Healthy-Living-V3/Eating-Disorders-The-physical-and-psychological-consequences-of-eating-disorders.html. Accessed on May 10, 2017.

"EDNOS: The Silent Killer." 2013. The Ranch. https://www.recoveryranch.com/articles/eating-disorders/ednos-the-silent-killer/. Accessed on May 14, 2017.

"The Effects of Bulimia on the Body." 2017. Healthline. http://www.healthline.com/health/bulimia/effects-on-body. Accessed on May 7, 2017.

"The Effects of Starvation on Behavior: Implications for Dieting and Eating Disorders." 2015. River Centre Clinic. http://river-centre.org/effects-starvation-behavior-implications-dieting-eating-disorders/. Accessed on May 11, 2017.

Ekern, Jacquelyn. 2017. "Binge Eating Disorder: Causes, Symptoms, Signs & Treatment Help." Eating Disorder Hope. https://www.eatingdisorderhope.com/information/

binge-eating-disorder#Signs-amp-Symptoms-of-Binge-Eating-Disorder. Accessed on May 7, 2017.

Feldman, Matthew B., and Ilan H. Meyer. 2007. "Eating Disorders in Diverse Lesbian, Gay, and Bisexual Populations." *International Journal of Eating Disorders*. 40(3): 218–226.

Ferguson, Christopher J., et al. 2014. "Concurrent and Prospective Analyses of Peer, Television and Social Media Influences on Body Dissatisfaction, Eating Disorder Symptoms and Life Satisfaction in Adolescent Girls." *Journal of Youth and Adolescence*. 43(1): 1–14.

Fielder-Jenks, Chelsea. 2017. "Mothers, Daughters, and Eating Disorders." Eating Disorder Hope. https://www.eating disorderhope.com/treatment-for-eating-disorders/family-role/mothers-daughters-and-eating-disorders. Accessed on May 23, 2017.

Fischer, Sarah, Monika Stojek, and Erin Hartzell. 2010. "Effects of Multiple Forms of Childhood Abuse and Adult Sexual Assault on Current Eating Disorder Symptoms." *Eating Behaviors*. 11(3): 190–192.

"Food and Diet." 2017. Harvard T. H. Chan School of Public Health. https://www.hsph.harvard.edu/obesity-prevention-source/obesity-causes/diet-and-weight/. Accessed on June 2, 2017.

"For Schools; In the Community; Sports & Fitness Industry." 2017. National Eating Disorders Collaboration. http://www.nedc.com.au/for-schools; http://www.nedc.com.au/in-the-community; http://www.nedc.com.au/sport-fitness-industry. Accessed on June 3, 2017.

Forney, K. Jean, Lauren A. Holland, and Pamela K. Keel. 2012. "Influence of Peer Context on the Relationship between Body Dissatisfaction and Eating Pathology in Women and Men." *International Journal of Eating Disorders*. 45(8): 982–989.

Francisco, Rita, Madalena Alarcão, and Isabel Narciso. 2012. "Aesthetic Sports as High-Risk Contexts for Eating Disorders—Young Elite Dancers and Gymnasts Perspectives." *The Spanish Journal of Psychology*. 15(1): 265–274.

Garner, David M. 1985. "Iatrogenesis in Anorexia Nervosa and Bulimia Nervosa." *International Journal of Eating Disorders*. 4(4): 701–726. https://www.researchgate.net/publication/229447793_Iatrogenesis_in_anorexia_nervosa_and_bulimia_nervosa. Accessed on June 5, 2017.

Garrido, Beatriz Jáuregui, and Ignacio Jáuregui Lobera. 2012. "Cardiovascular Complications in Eating Disorders." In *Relevant Topics in Eating Disorders* (online book). https://www.intechopen.com/books/relevant-topics-in-eating-disorders. Accessed on November 27, 2018.

Goldberg, Joseph. 2017. "Serious Health Problems Caused by Binge Eating." WebMD. http://www.webmd.com/mental-health/eating-disorders/binge-eating-disorder/health-problems-binge-eating#1. Accessed on May 12, 2017.

Gordon, Robert S. 1983. "An Operational Classification of Disease Prevention." *Public Health Reports*. 98(2): 107–109. https://www.ncbi.nlm.nih.gov/pmc/articles/PMC1424415/pdf/pubhealthrep00112-0005.pdf. Accessed on June 3, 2017.

Grewal, Seena, and Melissa Lieberman. 2016. "Avoidant/Restrictive Food Intake Disorder: Warning Signs and Symptoms." About Kids Health. https://www.aboutkidshealth.ca/Article?contentid=274&language=English. Accessed on November 27, 2018.

Halmi, Katherine A., et al. 2000. "Perfectionism in Anorexia Nervosa: Variation by Clinical Subtype, Obsessionality, and Pathological Eating Behavior." *American Journal of Psychiatry*. 157(11): 1799–1805. http://eatingdisorders.ucsd.edu/research/pub/imaging/doc/2000/halmi2000perfectionism.pdf. Accessed on May 19, 2017.

Hausenblas, Heather A., et al. 2012. "Media Effects of Experimental Presentation of the Ideal Physique on Eating Disorder Symptoms: A Meta-analysis of Laboratory Studies." *Clinical Psychology Review*. 33(1): 168–181. https://www .researchgate.net/publication/233900565_Media_effects_ of_experimental_presentation_of_the_ideal_physique_on_ eating_disorder_symptoms_A_meta-analysis_of_laboratory_ studies. Accessed on May 31, 2017.

Helfert, Susanne, and Petra Warschburger. 2013. "A Prospective Study on the Impact of Peer and Parental Pressure on Body Dissatisfaction in Adolescent Girls and Boys." *Body Image*. 8(2): 101–109.

Hinney, Anke, et al. 2006. "Genetic Risk Factors in Eating Disorders." *American Journal of PharmacoGenomics*. 4(4): 209–223.

"Home/Learn by Eating Disorder." 2016. National Eating Disorders Association. https://www.nationaleatingdisorders .org/learn/by-eating-disorder/. Accessed on May 6, 2017.

"Inpatient Program." 2017. The Center for Eating Disorders at Sheppard Pratt. https://eatingdisorder.org/treatment- and-support/levels-of-care/inpatient-program. Accessed on June 6, 2017.

Jade, Deanne. 2012. "The Effects of Under-Eating." National Centre for Eating Disorders. http://eating-disorders.org.uk/ information/the-effects-of-under-eating/. Accessed on May 10, 2017.

Jolly, Rhonda. 2011. "Marketing Obesity? Junk Food, Advertising, and Kids." Parliament of Australia. http:// www.aph.gov.au/About_Parliament/Parliamentary_ Departments/Parliamentary_Library/pubs/rp/ rp1011/11rp09#_Toc282609531. Accessed on June 2, 2017.

Kaye, Walter H., et al. 2004. "Comorbidity of Anxiety Disorders with Anorexia and Bulimia Nervosa." *American*

Journal of Psychiatry. 161(12): 2215–2221. http://
eatingdisorders.ucsd.edu/research/pub/imaging/doc/2004/
kaye2004comorbidity.pdf. Accessed on May 11, 2017.

Keith, S. W., et al. 2006. "Putative Contributors to the
Secular Increase in Obesity: Exploring the Roads Less
Traveled." *International Journal of Obesity.* 30(11):
1585–1594. http://www.andy.x10.bz/Pubs/Pub024.pdf.
Accessed on June 1, 2017.

Kong, S., and K. Bernstein. 2009. "Childhood Trauma as a
Predictor of Eating Psychopathology and Its Mediating
Variables in Patients with Eating Disorders." *Journal of
Clinical Nursing.* 18(13): 1897–1907.

Koven, Nancy S., and Alexandra W. Abry. 2015. "The
Clinical Basis of Orthorexia Nervosa: Emerging
Perspectives." *Neuropsychiatric Disease and Treatment.* 11:
385–394. https://www.ncbi.nlm.nih.gov/pmc/articles/
PMC4340368/. Accessed on May 8, 2017.

Kroon Van Diest, Ashley M., and Marisol Perez. 2012.
INTECH Open Access. http://cdn.intechopen.com/pdfs/
29060.pdf. Accessed on June 3, 2017.

Langmesser, Lisa, and Susan Verscheure. 2009. "Are Eating
Disorder Prevention Programs Effective?" *Journal of Athletic
Training.* 44(3): 304–305. https://www.ncbi.nlm.nih.gov/
pmc/articles/PMC2681220/. Accessed on June 4, 2017.

Le, Long Khanh-Dao, et al. 2017. "Prevention of Eating
Disorders: A Systematic Review and Meta-analysis." *Clinical
Psychology Review.* 53(7): 46–58.

Lee, Edward B., and Mark P. Mattson. 2014. "The
Neuropathology of Obesity: Insights from Human Disease."
Acta Neuropathologica. 127(1): 3–28. https://www.ncbi.nlm
.nih.gov/pmc/articles/PMC3880612/. Accessed on June 1,
2017.

Lentillon-Kaestner, V. 2015. "Male and Female Eating
Disorders in Fitness Sports." *Annals of Sports Medicine and*

Research. 2(6): 1039. https://www.jscimedcentral.com/
SportsMedicine/sportsmedicine-2-1039.pdf. Accessed on
May 25, 2017.

Levine, Michael P. 2015. "Does Prevention Work (and Is
This Even a Fair Question)?" Eating Disorders Resource
Catalog. https://www.edcatalogue.com/does-prevention-
work/. Accessed on June 4, 2017.

Levine, Michael P., and Sarah K. Murnen. 2009. " 'Everybody
Knows That Mass Media Are/Are Not [Pick One] a Cause
of Eating Disorders': A Critical Review of Evidence for
a Causal Link between Media, Negative Body Image,
and Disordered Eating in Females." *Journal of Social and
Clinical Psychology*. 28(1): 9–42. https://www.researchgate
.net/profile/Sarah_Murnen/publication/247839433_
Everybody_Knows_That_Mass_Media_areare_not_
pick_one_a_Cause_of_Eating_Disorders_A_Critical_
Review_of_Evidence_for_a_Causal_Link_Between_
Media_Negative_Body_Image_and_Disordered_
Eating_in_Females/links/0046352273f90464d9000000/
Everybody-Knows-That-Mass-Media-are-are-not-pick-
one-a-Cause-of-Eating-Disorders-A-Critical-Review-of-
Evidence-for-a-Causal-Link-Between-Media-Negative-
Body-Image-and-Disordered-Eating-in-Females.pdf.
Accessed on May 31, 2017.

Lionetti, Elena, et al. 2011. "Gastrointestinal Aspects of
Bulimia Nervosa." Intech Open Access. http://cdn
.intechopen.com/pdfs/21389.pdf. Accessed on May 12,
2017.

Litwack, Scott. D., et al. 2014. "Eating Disorder Symptoms
and Comorbid Psychopathology among Male and Female
Veterans." *General Hospital Psychiatry*. 36(4): 406–410.

Lucas, Valeri J. 2009. "Impact of Parenting Factors and
Personal Ego Development on Risk for Eating Disorders
among College Women." Marquette University
e-Publications. http://epublications.marquette.edu/cgi/

viewcontent.cgi?article=1075&context=dissertations_mu. Accessed on May 22, 2017.

Magallares, Alejandro. 2013. "Social Risk Factors Related to Eating Disorders in Women." *Revista Latinoamericana de Psicología.* 45(1): 147–154.

Magallares, Alejandro, and Jose Pais-Ribeiro. 2014. "Mental Health and Obesity: A Meta-analysis." *Applied Research in Quality of Life.* 9(2): 295–308. https://www.researchgate .net/publication/257691654_Mental_Health_and_ Obesity_A_Meta-Analysis#pf10. Accessed on June 7, 2017.

Malcolm, Allison, et al. 1997. "Rumination Syndrome." *Mayo Clinic Proceedings.* 72(7): 646–652. http://www.mayoclinic proceedings.org/article/S0025-6196(11)63571-4/fulltext. Accessed on May 13, 2017.

Mascolo, Margherita, et al. 2017. "Gastrointestinal Comorbidities Which Complicate the Treatment of Anorexia Nervosa." *Eating Disorders.* 25(2): 122–133.

McAllister, Emily J., et al. 2009. "Ten Putative Contributors to the Obesity Epidemic." *Critical Reviews in Food Science and Nutrition.* 49(10): 868–913. https://www.ncbi.nlm .nih.gov/pmc/articles/PMC2932668/. Accessed on June 1, 2017.

Meczekalski, Blazej, Agnieszka Podfigurna-Stopa, and Krzysztof Katulski. 2013. "Long-Term Consequences of Anorexia Nervosa." *Maturitas.* 75(3): 215–220.

Mehler, Philip, and Carrie Brown. 2015. "Anorexia Nervosa— Medical Complications." *Journal of Eating Disorders.* 3: 11. doi:10.1186/s40337-015-0040-8. https://jeatdisord.biomed central.com/articles/10.1186/s40337-015-0040-8. Accessed on May 9, 2017.

Micali, Nadia, et al. 2011. "Is Childhood OCD a Risk Factor for Eating Disorders Later in Life? A Longitudinal Study." *Psychological Medicine.* 41(12): 2507–2514. https://www

.researchgate.net/publication/51471184_Is_childhood_
OCD_a_risk_factor_for_eating_disorders_later_in_life_A_
longitudinal_study. Accessed on May 21, 2017.

Misra, Madhusmita, and Anne Klibanski. 2014. "Anorexia
Nervosa and Bone." *Journal of Endocrinology.* 221(3):
R163–R176. http://joe.endocrinology-journals.org/
content/221/3/R163.long. Accessed on May 9, 2017.

Mitchell, Karen S., et al. 2012. "Comorbidity of Partial
and Subthreshold PTSD among Men and Women with
Eating Disorders in the National Comorbidity Survey—
Replication Study." *International Journal of Eating
Disorders.* 45(3): 307–315.

Monteleone, Palmiero, and Mario Maj. 2013. "Dysfunctions
of Leptin, Ghrelin, BFNF and Endocannabinoids in Eating
Disorders: Beyond the Homeostatic Control of Food
Intake." *Psychoneuroendocrinology.* 38(3): 312–330.

Nattiv, Aurelia, et al. 2010. "The Female Athlete Triad."
Medscape. http://www.medscape.com/viewarticle/7170
52_1. Accessed on May 25, 2017.

Nicely, Terri A., et al. 2014. "Prevalence and Characteristics
of Avoidant/Restrictive Food Intake Disorder in a Cohort
of Young Patients in Day Treatment for Eating Disorders."
Journal of Eating Disorders. 2: 21. doi:10.1186/s40337-
014-0021-3. https://www.ncbi.nlm.nih.gov/pmc/articles/
PMC4145233/. Accessed on May 14, 2017.

Nilsson, Karin, et al. 2007. "Causes of Adolescent Onset
Anorexia Nervosa: Patient Perspectives." *Eating Disorders.*
15(2): 125–133. https://www.researchgate.net/profile/Karin_
Nilsson3/publication/6375172_Causes_of_Adolescent_
Onset_Anorexia_Nervosa_Patient_Perspectives/links/557ea
4bf08aeb61eae249ada.pdf. Accessed on May 19, 2017.

"Obesity and Sleep." 2017. National Sleep Foundation.
https://sleepfoundation.org/sleep-topics/obesity-and-sleep.
Accessed on June 2, 2017.

"Other Specified Feeding or Eating Disorders (OSFED)." 2017. Better Health Channel. https://www.betterhealth .vic.gov.au/health/healthyliving/other-specified-feeding-or- eating-disorders-osfed?viewAsPdf=true. Accessed on May 8, 2017.

Padez-Vieira, Francisca, and Pedro Afonso. 2016. "Sleep Disturbances in Anorexia Nervosa." *Advances in Eating Disorders*. 4(2): 176–188.

Patel, Priti, et al. 2002. "The Children of Mothers with Eating Disorders." *Clinical Child and Family Psychology Review*. 5(1): 1–19.

Patel, Sanjay R., and Frank B. Hu. 2008. "Short Sleep Duration and Weight Gain: A Systematic Review." *Obesity*. 16(3): 643–653.

Peterson, Carol, et al. 2016. "The Three-Legged Stool of Evidence-Based Practice in Eating Disorder Treatment: Research, Clinical, and Patient Perspectives." *BMC Medicine*. 14: 69. https://www.ncbi.nlm.nih.gov/pmc/articles/PMC48 32531/. Accessed on June 6, 2017.

Pike, Kathleen M., and Judith Rodin. 1991. "Mothers, Daughters, and Disordered Eating." *Journal of Abnormal Psychology*. 100(2): 198–204.

Pi-Sunyer, Xavier. 2015. "The Medical Risks of Obesity." *Postgraduate Medicine*. 121(6): 21–33. https://www.ncbi .nlm.nih.gov/pmc/articles/PMC2879283/. Accessed on June 7, 2017.

Polivy, Janet, and E. Peter Herman. 2002. "Causes of Eating Disorders." *Annual Review of Psychology*. 53: 187–214. https://is.muni.cz/el/1421/podzim2004/PSB_33/um/ eating_disorders.pdf. Accessed on May 20, 2017.

Poyastro Pinheiro, Andrea, Tammy Root, and Cynthia M Bulik. 2009. "The Genetics of Anorexia Nervosa: Current Findings and Future Perspectives." *International Journal of Child and Adolescent Health*. 2(2): 153–164.

"Prevalence in Men." 2017. National Eating Disorders Association. https://www.nationaleatingdisorders.org/research-males-and-eating-disorders. Accessed on May 17, 2017.

Raven, Sarah. 2016. "Iatrogenic Effects." Dr. Sarah Ravin. http://www.blog.drsarahravin.com/eating-disorders/iatrogenic-effects/. Accessed on June 5, 2017.

Russell, Christopher J., and Pamela K. Keel. 2002. "Homosexuality as a Specific Risk Factor for Eating Disorders in Men." *International Journal of Eating Disorders.* 31(3): 300–306.

Rutsztein, Guillermina, M. Light Scappatura, and Brenda Murawski. 2014. "Perfectionism and Low Self-Esteem across the Continuum of Eating Disorders in Adolescent Girls from Buenos Aires." *Mexican Journal of Eating Disorders.* 5(1): 39–49. http://www.sciencedirect.com/science/article/pii/S2007152314703751. Accessed on May 20, 2017. Original in Spanish, translatable to English.

Sachs, Katherine V., et al. 2016. "Cardiovascular Complications of Anorexia Nervosa: A Systematic Review." *International Journal of Eating Disorders.* 49(3): 238–248.

Sanci, Lena, et al. 2008. "Childhood Sexual Abuse and Eating Disorders in Females: Findings from the Victorian Adolescent Health Cohort Study." *Archives of Pediatric and Adolescent Medicine.* 162(3): 261–267.

Sansone, Randy A., and Lori A. Sansone. 2010. "Personality Disorders as Risk Factors for Eating Disorders: Clinical Implications." *Nutrition in Clinical Practice.* 25(2): 116–121.

Sassaroli, Sandra, Marcello Gallucci, and Giovanni Maria Ruggiero. 2008. "Low Perception of Control as a Cognitive Factor of Eating Disorders. Its Independent Effects on Measures of Eating Disorders and Its Interactive Effects with Perfectionism and Self-Esteem." *Journal of Behavior Therapy and Experimental Psychiatry.* 39(4): 467–488.

Schmidt, Randy. 2010. "Karen Carpenter's Tragic Story." *Guardian*. https://www.theguardian.com/books/2010/oct/24/karen-carpenter-anorexia-book-extract. Accessed on May 9, 2017.

Scott-Van Zeeland, A. A., et al. 2014. "Evidence for the Role of EPHX2 Gene Variants in Anorexia Nervosa." *Molecular Psychiatry*. 19: 724–732. https://www.ncbi.nlm.nih.gov/pmc/articles/PMC3852189/. Accessed on June 5, 2017.

Segel, Carol M., ed. 2011. *Childhood Obesity: Risk Factors, Health Effects, and Prevention*. Hauppauge, NY: Nova Science.

"Selecting a Treatment Center for Your Loved One." 2017. National Eating Disorder Association. https://www.national eatingdisorders.org/selecting-treatment-center-your-loved-one. Accessed on June 5, 2017.

Shaw, Heather, Eric Stice, and Carolyn Black Becker. 2009. "Preventing Eating Disorders." *Child and Adolescent Psychiatric Clinics of North America*. 18(1): 199–207. https://www.ncbi.nlm.nih.gov/pmc/articles/PMC2938770/. Accessed on June 4, 2017.

Sidiropoulos, Michael. 2007. "Anorexia Nervosa: The Physiological Consequences of Starvation and the Need for Primary Prevention Efforts." *McGill Journal of Medicine*. 10(1): 20–25. https://www.ncbi.nlm.nih.gov/pmc/articles/PMC2323541/. Accessed on May 9, 2017.

Smith, Pauline M., and Alastair V. Ferguson. 2008. "Neurophysiology of Hunger and Satiety." *Developmental Disabilities Research Reviews*. 14(2): 96–104. https://www.researchgate.net/publication/51419870_Neurophysiology_of_hunger_and_satiety. Accessed on May 30, 2017.

Stern, Judith S., and Alexandra Kazaks. 2015. *Obesity: A Reference Handbook*, 2nd ed. Santa Barbara, CA: ABC-CLIO.

Stice, Eric, and Kyle Burger. 2015. "Dieting as a Risk Factor for Eating Disorders." In Linda Smolak and Michael P.

Levine, eds. *The Wiley Handbook of Eating Disorders*, chapter 24, 312–323. Chichester: John Wiley & Sons.

Stice, Eric, Jennifer Maxfield, and Tony Wells. 2003. "Adverse Effects of Social Pressure to Be Thin on Young Women: An Experimental Investigation of the Effects of 'Fat Talk.'" *International Journal of Eating Disorders*. 34(1): 108–117. http://onlinelibrary.wiley.com/doi/10.1002/eat.10171/pdf. Accessed on May 24, 2017.

Stice, Eric, and Heather Shaw. 2004. "Eating Disorder Prevention Programs: A Meta-analytic Review." *Psychological Bulletin*. 130(2): 206–227.

Stice, Eric, and Kathryn Whitenton. 2002. "Risk Factors for Body Dissatisfaction in Adolescent Girls: A Longitudinal Investigation." *Developmental Psychology*. 38(5): 669–678. http://www.ori.org/files/Static%20Page%20Files/ SticeWhitenton02.pdf. Accessed on May 17, 2017.

Stiegler, Lillian. 2005. "Understanding Pica Behavior." *Focus on Autism and Other Developmental Disabilities*. 20(1): 27–38. https://www.researchgate.net/publication/2459236 74_Understanding_Pica_Behavior. Accessed on May 13, 2017.

Stitt, Natalie. 2012. "The Experiences of Parents with an Eating Disorder." Monash University. http://www.copmi .net.au/images/pdf/Research/Clearinghouse/parent-experiences-of-eating-disorder.pdf. Accessed on May 23, 2017.

Striegel-Moore, Ruth, and Cynthia Bulk. 2007. "Risk Factors for Eating Disorders." *American Psychologist*. 62(3): 181–198. https://www.researchgate.net/publication/6359 966_Risk_Factors_for_Eating_Disorders. Accessed on May 16, 2017.

Strober, Michael. 2004. "Managing the Chronic, Treatment-Resistant Patient with Anorexia Nervosa." *International Journal of Eating Disorders*. 36(3): 245–255.

Strober, Michael, and Laura L. Humphrey. 1987 "Familial Contributions to the Etiology and Course of Anorexia Nervosa and Bulimia." *Journal of Consulting and Clinical Psychology.* 55(5): 654–659.

Strober, Michael, et al. 2000. "Controlled Family Study of Anorexia Nervosa and Bulimia Nervosa: Evidence of Shared Liability and Transmission of Partial Syndromes." *American Journal of Psychiatry.* 157(3): 393–401.

Strumia, Renata, ed. 2013. *Eating Disorders and the Skin.* Heidelberg: Springer.

"Symptoms of Demonic Bondage." 2017. http://www.warriors 4thelamb.com/index.php?page_id=34. Accessed on May 18, 2017.

Tafà, Mimma, et al. 2017. "Female Adolescents with Eating Disorders, Parental Psychopathological Risk and Family Functioning." *Journal of Child and Family Studies.* 26(1): 28–39.

Tangney, June P., Roy F. Baumeister, and Angie Luzio Boone. 2004. "High Self-Control Predicts Good Adjustment, Less Pathology, Better Grades, and Interpersonal Success." *Journal of Personality.* 72(2): 271–324.

Tetyana. 2012. "When Clinicians Do More Harm Than Good—Part 2 (Risks Associated with Treatment)." Science of Eating Disorders. http://www.scienceofeds .org/2012/07/12/when-clinicians-do-more-harm-than-good-part-2-iatrogenic-factors/. Accessed on June 5, 2017.

Thein-Nissenbaum, Jill. 2013. "Long Term Consequences of the Female Athlete." *Maturitas.* 75(2): 107–112.

Throckmorton, Warren. 2016. "Mark Driscoll Takes on Anorexia: Might Be Demonic." Patheos. http://www.patheos .com/blogs/warrenthrockmorton/2016/05/16/mark-driscoll-takes-on-anorexia-might-be-demonic/. Accessed on May 18, 2017.

Tiggemann, Marika, and Melissa Raven. 1998. "Dimensions of Control in Bulimia and Anorexia Nervosa: Internal Control, Desire for Control, or Fear of Losing Self-Control?" *Eating Disorders.* 6(1): 65–72.

Tomba, Elena, et al. 2014. "Psychological Well-Being in Out-Patients with Eating Disorders: A Controlled Study." *International Journal of Eating Disorders.* 47(3): 252–258.

Tozzi, Federica, et al. 2003. "Causes and Recovery in Anorexia Nervosa: The Patient's Perspective." *International Journal of Eating Disorders.* 33(2): 143–154. https://www .researchgate.net/publication/10873309_Causes_and_ recovery_in_anorexia_nervosa_The_patient's_perspective. Accessed on May 19, 2017.

"Treatment Settings and Levels of Care." 2017. National Eating Disorders Association. https://www.nationaleating disorders.org/treatment-settings-and-levels-care. Accessed on June 5, 2017.

"Understanding Anorexia Treatment: What to Expect during the First Week in Residential Treatment." 2015. Eating Disorder Hope. https://www.eatingdisorderhope.com/information/ anorexia/understanding-anorexia-treatment-what-to-expect-during-the-first-week-in-residential-treatment. Accessed on June 6, 2017.

"Understanding the Warning Signs." 2015. National Eating Disorders Collaboration. http://www.nedc.com.au/recog nise-the-warning-signs. Accessed on May 6, 2017.

Valena, V., and W. G. Young. 2002. "Dental Erosion Patterns from Intrinsic Acid Regurgitation and Vomiting." *Australian Dental Journal.* 47(2): 106–115.

Vorstman, Jacob A. S., and Roel A. Ophoff. 2013. "Genetic Causes of Developmental Disorders." *Current Opinion in Neurology.* 26(2): 128–136.

Wang, K., et al. 2010. "A Genome-Wide Association Study on Common SNPs and Rare CNVs in Anorexia Nervosa."

Molecular Psychiatry. 16: 949–959. https://www.nature
.com/mp/journal/v16/n9/full/mp2010107a.html. Accessed
on May 29, 2017.

"Warning Signs and Symptoms [for ARFID]." 2016. National
Eating Disorders Association. https://www.nationaleating
disorders.org/learn/by-eating-disorder/arfid/warning-signs-
symptoms. Accessed on May 8, 2017.

Warren, Michelle P. 2011. "Endocrine Manifestations of
Eating Disorders." *Journal of Endocrinological Metabolism.*
96(2): 333–343.

Weaver, Jolanta U. 2008. "Classical Endocrine Diseases
Causing Obesity." *Frontiers of Hormone Research.* 36:
212–228.

Welch, Elisabeth, and Ata Ghaderi. 2012. "Eating Disorders
and Self-Esteem." In Anna-Karin Andershed, ed. *Girls at
Risk: Swedish Longitudinal Research on Adjustment.* New
York: Springer, 35–56.

"What Is OSFED?" 2017. National Eating Disorders
Collaborative. http://www.nedc.com.au/files/Resources/
OSFED%20Fact%20Sheet.pdf. Accessed on May 8, 2017.

"What People with Anorexia Nervosa Need to Know about
Osteoporosis." 2016. NIH Osteoporosis and Related Bone
Diseases National Resource Center. https://www.niams
.nih.gov/Health_Info/Bone/Osteoporosis/Conditions_
Behaviors/anorexia_nervosa.asp. Accessed on May 9, 2017.

Wilksch, Simon M. 2014. "Where Did Universal Eating
Disorder Prevention Go?" *Eating Disorders.* 22(2): 184–192.
https://www.researchgate.net/publication/259446167_
Where_Did_Universal_Eating_Disorder_Prevention_Go.
Accessed on June 3, 2017.

Woodside, D. Blake, et al. 2002. "Personality, Perfectionism,
and Attitudes toward Eating in Parents of Individuals
with Eating Disorders." *International Journal of Eating
Disorders.* 31(3): 290–299. https://www.researchgate.net/

publication/11444200_Personality_perfectionism_and_
attitudes_toward_eating_in_parents_of_individuals_with_
eating_disorders. Accessed on May 22, 2017.

Yahalom, Malka, et al. 2013. "The Significance of Bradycardia
in Anorexia Nervosa." *International Journal of Angiology.*
22(2): 83–94. https://www.ncbi.nlm.nih.gov/pmc/articles/
PMC3709923/. Accessed on May 9, 2017.

Yeager, Kimberly K., et al. 1993. "The Female Athlete Triad:
Disordered Eating, Amenorrhea, Osteoporosis." *Medicine &
Science in Sports & Exercise.* 25(7): 775–777.

Zepf, Bill. 2004. "Metabolic Abnormalities in Bulimia
Nervosa." *American Family Physician.* 69(6): 1530–1532.
http://www.aafp.org/afp/2004/0315/p1530.html. Accessed
on May 12, 2017.

Zickgraf, Hana F., Marting E. Franklin, and Paul Rozin.
2016. "Adult Picky Eaters with Symptoms of Avoidant/
Restrictive Food Intake Disorder: Comparable Distress and
Comorbidity but Different Eating Behaviors Compared
to Those with Disordered Eating Symptoms." *Journal of
Eating Disorders.* 4: 26. doi:10.1186/s40337-016-0110-6.
https://www.ncbi.nlm.nih.gov/pmc/articles/PMC5086050/.
Accessed on May 8, 2017.

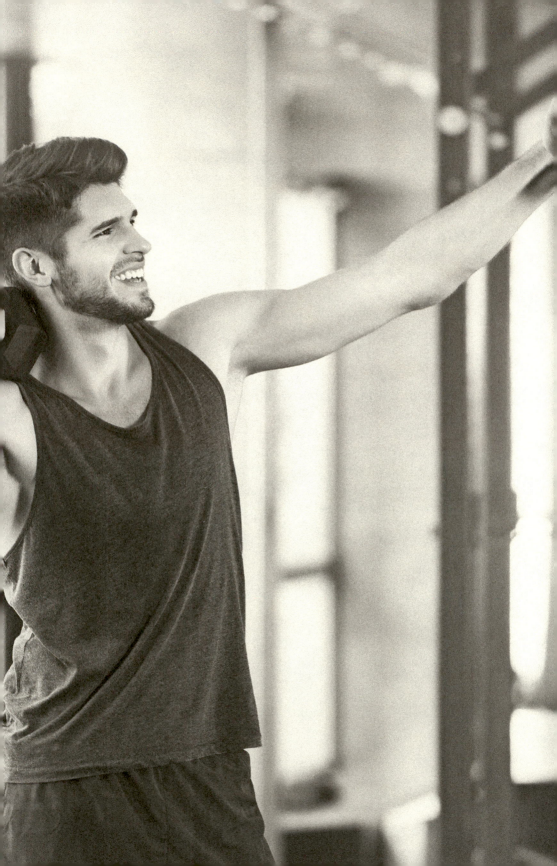

Eating disorders is a subject that provokes a variety of opinions. This chapter provides an opportunity for individuals with an interest in the topic to present their own views on some specific aspect of the subject.

Social Media and Relationship between Body Image and Eating Disorders
Jac Julien

How much time do you spend on social media such as Facebook, Instagram, and YouTube? What happens when you view this social media and make comparisons about yourself to others that you see? Social media use and engagement is a growing influence on body image and dissatisfaction leading to eating disorders. Research is currently exploring the relationship between social media use and body image issues (e.g., the thinness ideal, body image dissatisfaction) that are related to eating disorders. There is even a suggestion that for adolescents the relationship between eating disorders and social media viewing is as strong as or stronger than for other types of passive media such as television (Cohen and Blaszczynski 2015, 4). In fact, research (Bair et al. 2012, 400) suggests that women

---

A young man takes a selfie while lifting weights at the gym. Social media provides new forums for weight comparison and obsession. (Vadymvdrobot/ Dreamstime.com)

who used the Internet more frequently were more likely to develop disordered eating.

Of critical importance in the relationship among social media use, body concerns, and eating disorders are the time spent on and the type of interactions that a person has on social media sites. Research (Holland and Tiggemann 2016, 106) suggests that the time spent using and investment in Facebook are associated with users feeling more body conscious and having more bodily shame. Those who wrote statuses that were slanted to receive negative feedback reported higher concerns with body shape, eating, and weight (Holland and Tiggemann 2016, 106). Mabe (Mabe et al. 2014, 520) found that simply spending 20 minutes on Facebook resulted in higher concern about a person's weight and shape and that the amount of time a user spent on Facebook related to higher rates of disordered eating.

In addition, the way in which a person compares himself or herself to others when viewing social media correlates to eating disorder concerns. Simply put, sharing more photos on Facebook is related to higher levels of the thin ideal (Holland and Tiggemann 2016, 106). Social media users were more likely to rate their bodies as worse than celebrities and close and distant friends. The more time spent in comparison to peers, the more a person experienced body dissatisfaction (Fardouly and Vartanian 2014, 86). Facebook users who engaged in more social comparison and elicited negative feedback from others were likely to experience an increase in bulimic symptoms and eating disorder pathology (Cohen and Blaszczynski 2015, 4; Smith et al. 2013, 239). Furthermore, Facebook users who more often engaged with others, by liking or commenting on photos, showed higher comparisons to others' appearance (Holland and Tiggemann 2016, 106). Simply viewing others' photos on Facebook, with no interaction, also related to internalization of the thin ideal, drive for thinness and weight dissatisfaction (Holland and Tiggemann 2016, 106).

Not only did use of social media and comparisons with others result in short-term comparisons and body image issues, but also there is some suggestion that those issues can lead to long-term body image disturbances and eating issues. Facebook users who wrote more revealing status updates and received negative feedback were more likely to be eating more and concerned about their body shape and weight at a four-week follow-up (Holland and Tiggemann 2016, 106). Smith et al. (2013, 239) also found that Facebook users who did more social comparison and received negative comments on status updates were likely to engage in overeating and have an increase in bulimic symptoms at a four-week follow-up. Holland and Tiggemann (2016, 106) suggest the more time a person spends on social media may predict body image and eating concerns up to 18 months later.

One caveat of the current research is that most has been completed using Facebook. More research should be conducted to determine if other types of social media result in the same types of issues related to body dissatisfaction and eating disorders. However, given the similar interactive nature across all social media platforms and the research that has been conducted on social media aside from Facebook, it seems that the influence on body image and disordered eating crosses social media platforms.

Social media appears to be a stronger influencer on users in relation to their body image and disordered eating than more passive media such as television and magazines. The more time and interaction a user has on social media leads to more distorted thinking about one's body and the development of disordered eating. Simply using social media may lead to comparisons with others and become a significant factor in issues of concern over weight, the thin ideal, body shape, symptoms of bulimia, and eating disorders. The influence of social media use on a person certainly is short term but may also carry over into long-term comparisons.

Those who engage in social media, particularly those who are at risk for body dissatisfaction and eating disorders, may want to limit the amount of time they spend on social media sites, in one sitting as well as in general. Comparisons to others on social media appears to be a major factor for those at risk of an eating disorder. It is wise to keep in mind that on social media people portray the best facets of their life. Social media users should think about the types of updates they are making and focus on gaining more positive feedback from others. It should be of note that the effects of social media use as it impacts body dissatisfaction and disordered eating may carry over long after the user has logged off.

References

Bair, Carrie E., et al. 2012. "Does the Internet Function Like Magazines? An Exploration of Image-Focused Media, Eating Pathology, and Body Dissatisfaction." *Eating Behaviors*. 13(4): 398–401.

Cohen, Rachel, and Alex Blaszczynski. 2015. "Comparative Effects of Facebook and Conventional Media on Body Image Dissatisfaction." *Journal of Eating Disorders*. 3(1): 1–11.

Fardouly, Jasmine, and Lenny R. Vartanian. 2015. "Negative Comparisons about One's Appearance Mediate the Relationship between Facebook Usage and Body Image Concerns." *Body Image*. 12: 82–88.

Holland, Grace, and Marika Tiggemann. 2016. "A Systematic Review of the Impact of the Use of Social Networking Sites on Body Image and Disordered Eating Outcomes." *Body Image*. 17: 100–110.

Mabe, Annalise G., et al. 2014. "Do You 'Like' My Photo? Facebook Use Maintains Eating Disorder Risk." *International Journal of Eating Disorders*. 47: 516–523.

Smith, April R., et al. 2013. "Status Update: Maladaptive Facebook Usage Predicts Increases in Body Dissatisfaction and Bulimic Symptoms." *Journal of Affective Disorders.* 149: 235–240.

Jacqueline Julien is a Well-Life Coach and creator of The Empowered Life Diet. She helps women overcome their emotional eating issues through living their empowered life. She holds a PsyD in clinical psychology. She may be reached at www.jacjulien.com.

What Goes on in the Brain of an Anorexic?
David L. Levine

Anorexia nervosa is an eating disorder that is characterized by self-starvation and excessive weight loss. People with anorexia place a high value on controlling their weight and shape. They have both an intense fear of gaining weight and a distorted perception of body weight leading to extreme efforts to control calorie intake by vomiting after eating or by misusing laxatives, diet aids, diuretics, or enemas that tend to significantly interfere with activities in their lives (Anorexia Nervosa 2017).

Approximately 1 percent of American women will suffer anorexia in their lifetime, according to the National Association of Anorexia Nervosa and Associated Disorders (Eating Disorder Statistics 2017). The association also notes that 50–80 percent of the risk for anorexia and bulimia is genetic; 33–50 percent of anorexia patients have a mood disorder, such as depression; and about 50 percent of people with anorexia suffer from anxiety disorders such as obsessive-compulsive disorder and social phobia. Anorexia is most often seen in young women who feel that they need to stay thin to be attractive, but it can affect the elderly as well.

We are fortunate to live in a country where people generally understand that depression and obsessive-compulsive disorder are mental illnesses and not a weakness of character. And this is important. Mental illness was not seen as a problem of the brain but as a personality defect that must be hidden. Many people who sought help from psychiatrists would pay in cash or not put claims through insurance out of fear of embarrassment or being passed over by promotions by their employers. And as late as the 1950s–1960s, autism was blamed as being caused by indifferent, cold mothers, aka "the refrigerator mom" (Laidler 2004).

It is easy to think that females who obsessively watch their diet want to be fashionably thin as the models they see on magazines. (Although there are male anorexics, anorexia is predominantly seen in women.) It would also be easy to blame anorexia as a reaction to societal pressures to attract a boyfriend or husband or to the obesity epidemic in America.

And although societal factors play a role in weight, people with anorexia have intense fears of becoming fat and see themselves as fat even when they are very thin. It is a true mental illness. In fact, studies have shown anorexia to carry a six-fold increased risk of death, greater than that of major depression, bipolar disorder, and schizophrenia. And scientists had observed that anorexia often ran in families like schizophrenia, depression, and anxiety disorders.

A 2017 study led by researchers at the University of North Carolina School of Medicine identified the first genetic locus for anorexia and found that there may also be metabolic underpinnings to the disease. The study, published in the *American Journal of Psychiatry*, involved a genome-wide analysis of DNA from 3,495 individuals with anorexia and 10,982 without anorexia (Duncan et al. 2017).

An international collaboration of scientists found that many people who suffer from anorexia nervosa have mutated DNA on a particular chromosome. The researchers found that anorexia was partly genetic and the risk of developing an eating disorder could be passed onto children. Lead researcher Cynthia Bulik, of the University of North Carolina, said about the study: "Anorexia nervosa was significantly genetically correlated with neuroticism and schizophrenia, supporting the idea that anorexia is indeed a psychiatric illness." "Unexpectedly," Dr. Bulik said, "we also found strong genetic correlations with various metabolic features including body composition (BMI) and insulin–glucose metabolism. This finding encourages us to look more deeply at how metabolic factors increase the risk for anorexia nervosa" (For Anorexia Nervosa, Researchers Implicate Genetic Locus on Chromosome 12 2017).

This research adds to previous research done at the California Institute of Technology (Caltech), which identified a population of neurons in the central amygdala region of the brain that controls feeding behavior. The research team, whose results were published in *Nature Neuroscience*, found that they could manipulate the neurons in the mouse brain and turn off the brain's desire for food. They noted that identifying these neurons might lead to an inhibitory control of feeding and someday lead to better treatments for eating disorders, such as anorexia or bulimia, or for obesity (Cai et al. 2014).

A study conducted by researchers at Columbia University Medical Center, New York State Psychiatric Institute, the Mortimer B. Zuckerman Mind Brain Behavior Institute, and New York University found that the brains of people with anorexia were similar to the brains of people who suffered from substance abuse or were addicted to gambling. The researchers knew that people with anorexia desire low-calorie, low-fat food, regardless of the individuals' desire for change. However, the brain mechanisms underlying this behavior have never been understood.

The researchers used functional magnetic resonance imaging to monitor women with anorexia nervosa and a control group of healthy individuals while they made a series of choices about what food to eat. The individuals with anorexia nervosa consistently chose fewer high-fat foods. The researchers found that the brain regions they used to make those choices were different from the healthy controls. For the individuals with anorexia nervosa, choices about what to eat were associated with activation in the dorsal striatum, a brain region known to be related to habitual control of actions. In addition, activation in fronto-striatal brain circuits during the experiment predicted how many calories they chose to consume in a meal the following day. This study is the first to link abnormalities in brain activity with restrictive food choice, the main symptom of anorexia nervosa (Foerde et al. 2015).

It is natural to think that people who are dangerously thin would notice and seek medical attention and gain weight. But most do not. One of the reasons is that anorexics have a disconnection from their own body. "When anorexics look in the mirror they think they are larger than they actually are. Their brains retain old images and the anorexic sees a perception of a larger self that is out of date," according to Jane Aspell, senior lecturer in psychology at Anglia Ruskin University. Aspell and her colleagues generated an "out-of-body experience" through the visual projection of human heartbeats. The goal was to make the volunteers feel as if they were inhabiting an image of their own body, which was projected 2 meters away from their actual bodies. The researchers synchronized the virtual image with the participants' heartbeats in real time, causing the subjects to have a strong identification with their body "double" and making them feel that they were closer to the virtual image body than to their own bodies (Aspell et al. 2013).

"This research demonstrates that the experience of one's self can be altered when presented with information about the internal state of one's body, such as a heartbeat," Dr. Aspell said. "This experiment could be adapted to help people 'reconnect' with their current physical appearance and help them realize what the 'real me' actually looks like." Aspell noted that this type of technology might help the brain "update" its representation of the body after it heals and changes in recovery.

With a greater understanding of what occurs in the brains of people with anorexia, and perhaps with the aid of avatars to help them to see themselves as they are in real time, there is new hope for people who suffer from an ailment that is difficult to treat and a challenge to the anorexics, their family, and the doctors who treat them.

References

"Anorexia Nervosa." 2017. Mayo Clinic. http://www.mayo clinic.org/diseases-conditions/anorexia/home/ovc-2017 9508. Accessed May 17, 2017.

Aspell, J. E., et al. 2013. "Turning Body and Self Inside Out: Visualized Heartbeats Alter Bodily Self-Consciousness and Tactile Perception." *Psychological Science.* 24(12): 2445–2453.

Cai, H., et al. 2014. "Central Amygdala PKC-δ(+) Neurons Mediate the Influence of Multiple Anorexigenic Signals." *Nature Neuroscience.* 17(9): 1240–1248.

Duncan, L., et al. 2017. "Significant Locus and Metabolic Genetic Correlations Revealed in Genome-Wide Association Study of Anorexia Nervosa." *American Journal of Psychiatry.* http://dx.doi.org/10.1176/appi.ajp.2017.16121402. Accessed on May 17, 2017.

"Eating Disorder Statistics." 2017. National Association of Anorexia Nervosa and Associated Disorders. http://www .anad.org/get-information/about-eating-disorders/eating-disorders-statistics/. Accessed May 17, 2017.

Foerde, Karin, et al. 2015. "Neural Mechanisms Supporting Maladaptive Food Choices in Anorexia Nervosa." *Nature Neuroscience.* 18(11): 1571–1573.

"For Anorexia Nervosa, Researchers Implicate Genetic Locus on Chromosome 12." Medical Xpress. https://medicalxpress .com/news/2017-05-anorexia-nervosa-implicate-genetic-locus.html#jCp. Accessed on May 17, 2017.

Laidler, James R. 2004. "The 'Refrigerator Mother' Hypothesis of Autism." Autism Watch. https://www.autism-watch.org/causes/rm.shtml. Accessed May 17, 2017.

David L. Levine is cochairman of Science Writers in New York and a member of the National Association of Science Writers and the Association of Healthcare Journalists. He writes for The New York Times, *Reuters Health,* Scientific American Mind, Nature Medicine, *the* Los Angeles Times, Nautilus, *and the* Smithsonian. *He was a contributing editor at* Physician's Weekly *for 10 years. He served as director of media relations at the American Cancer Society and as senior director of communications at the NYC Health and Hospitals Corp. He has a BA and an MA from The Johns Hopkins University.*

Picky Eating or an Eating Disorder? Spotting the Newest Eating Disorder in Children
Kimberley Peterman

Growing up, I made it very well known that I did not care for eating certain things. Nothing could touch; the mixing of textures made me gag. Even vaguely spicy foods would be spit out as soon as they touched my tongue. I would eat only certain fruits and vegetables because of how they felt on my tongue. Nearly a decade later, my youngest brother was even worse, not wanting to eat almost anything.

Thankfully, our parents were able to feed us so that we could maintain a healthy body weight, and we grew out of most of our picky habits, like most kids. However, there are those children whose picky tastes impede them from eating a healthy amount altogether, thus preventing them from reaching a healthy weight. Those children are suffering from avoidant/restrictive food intake disorder (ARFID).

ARFID is a disorder that was introduced in the fifth edition of the *Diagnostic and Statistical Manual of Mental Disorders.* A new eating disorder, it affects those who exhibit many of the traditional symptoms of an eating disorder, such as extreme weight loss and nutritional deficiencies, but with no skewed body image (Norris et al. 2013, 496). The main effect of its conception has been a decrease in the diagnoses for eating disorder not otherwise specified (Ornstein et al. 2013, 304). However, this newness means that it is not well known, there are not many statistics on it, and the symptoms can be difficult to identify. As such, many studies have come out in recent years, which retrospectively examined statistics of eating disorders to diagnose previous cases that exhibited symptoms of ARFID.

Statistically, ARFID occurs more frequently in boys than do other eating disorders and, on average, in a younger age group. One study found that 21 percent of those suffering from ARFID were male and 41 percent were below the age of 12, while only 8 percent of those suffering from anorexia were male and 2.8 percent were below 12 years (Norris et al. 2013, 496). This makes sense since most children wouldn't care about body image. However, because so many children go through a phase where they don't want to eat certain foods to begin with, it may be difficult for parents to identify if their child is just a picky eater or suffers from ARFID.

While ARFID is characterized by an aversion to food, the condition could stem from extreme concerns about food choices, a general aversion to food, a fear of eating in front of others, or even a fear of choking or vomiting as a result of eating. The main symptoms that should signal parents that their child might have the condition are a severe drop in weight or, particularly in the case of children, a failure to gain weight or grow. Other signs can be extreme nutritional deficiencies that require supplements to make up the lack of nutrients (Niego 2017). If these symptoms coincide with the child's pickiness rather than an obsession with weight or appearance, then their child may have ARFID.

This combination of symptoms may seem easy to spot and, once the general symptoms of an eating disorder appear, it should be. Yet parents would want to prevent their child from reaching the point of being underweight. The best way to identify this problem is to make sure the child is consuming enough calories and nutrients for his or her weight and age. This information is available from one's pediatrician or programs like MyPlate, created by the U.S. Department of Agriculture ("Choose MyPlate" 2017). If the child's preferences, anxieties, or other psychological aversions to eating are preventing him or her from eating a healthy amount, then the child's parents should consult a doctor. Thankfully, ARFID is just as treatable as any eating disorder by specialists, so once diagnosed, children can recover.

Almost all children go through phases of picky eating. However, this new disorder could lead some parents to diagnose children with the condition prematurely or to spot the signs too late. By monitoring a child's food intake, one could prevent a child from suffering from malnutrition or malnourishment as the result of the eating disorder.

References

"Choose MyPlate." 2017. U.S. Department of Agriculture. https://www.choosemyplate.gov/. Accessed on May 20, 2017.

Niego, Sara. 2017. "Signs That a Child Is More Than Just A Picky Eater: What Every Parent Needs to Know about ARFID." Greenwich Free Press. https://greenwichfreepress .com/health/signs-that-a-child-is-more-than-just-a-picky-eater-what-every-parent-needs-to-know-about-arfid-81310/. Accessed on May 20, 2017.

Norris, Mark L., et al. 2013. "Exploring Avoidant/Restrictive Food Intake Disorder in Eating Disordered Patients: A Descriptive Study." *International Journal of Eating Disorders*. 47(5): 495–499.

Ornstein, Rollyn M., et al. 2013. "Distribution of Eating Disorders in Children and Adolescents Using the Proposed DSM-5 Criteria for Feeding and Eating Disorders." *Journal of Adolescent Health*. 53(2): 303–305.

Kimberley Peterman is a rising senior at Rutgers University. With four-and-a-half years of research experience, she has two previously published papers in cellular biology and epigenetics and has also presented a paper at the Harry Potter Conference at Chestnut Hill College. In her free time she enjoys blogging, reading, and singing, as well as learning new languages, history, pop culture, and the stories of all types of people.

Debunking Common Myths about Eating Disorders
Jennifer Rollin

"I can't possibly have anorexia, because I'm in my 50s. That's something that teenagers get!" she exclaimed. This kind of sentiment is unfortunately far too common for those struggling with eating disorders, who may not fit the narrow stereotypical mold of "what someone with an eating disorder looks like."

Anorexia nervosa is the deadliest mental illness. However, unfortunately eating disorders are often highly stigmatized, stereotyped, and generally misunderstood. As an eating disorder therapist in private practice, in Rockville, Maryland, I have seen the negative implications that stigma and stereotypes can have on individuals who are struggling with eating disorders.

It is important to debunk common myths to generate a better understanding of eating disorders, for those who are struggling, loved ones, and treatment professionals. Through education and raising awareness, we can encourage individuals who are suffering with eating disorders to seek life-saving treatment.

Myths about Eating Disorders

1. Eating disorders are caused by vanity or thin models in magazines.

People who struggle with eating disorders are not "vain" or "shallow." While often individuals with eating disorders might present with concerns about weight and food, this is simply the way that the symptoms of illness manifest.

The reality is that eating disorders are serious mental illnesses, which, research suggests, are caused by a combination of genetic, temperamental, and psychological factors, which are then triggered by environmental stressors.

While the media and diet culture may trigger someone with the underlying genetic, temperamental, and psychological factors, they are certainty not the sole cause that contributes to an individual developing an eating disorder.

2. Eating disorders affect only young, Caucasian females.

Eating disorders do not discriminate based on age, gender, socioeconomic status, or race. There is a common misperception that eating disorders affect only young, Caucasian females, as this is primarily what is displayed in the media. However, I have seen clients of a wide variety of ages, races, and ethnicities, as well as males, females, and transgender individuals, in my eating disorder therapy practice.

Further, individuals who do not fit the narrow mold of what people stereotype someone with an eating disorder to "look like" may not seek treatment due to shame, stigma, and denial of their illness. Thus, current statistics may not be a reliable source of data regarding the gender, ethnicity, race, and so on of individuals who are struggling with eating disorders.

3. You can tell who is struggling with an eating disorder based on his or her appearance.

Eating disorders are one of the few mental illnesses, where people falsely believe that you can judge someone's struggle or "level of suffering" based on his or her physical appearance.

It's important to note that you cannot tell who is struggling with an eating disorder based on his or her appearance. Some individuals struggling with eating disorders may "appear healthy" but be quite mentally and physically unwell.

In addition, there is a common misconception that individuals struggling with eating disorders always appear emaciated or even "thin." However, the reality is that someone can be severely struggling with an eating disorder across the weight spectrum.

The myth that one must appear "emaciated" or "thin" to be struggling with an eating disorder may prevent people from seeking the help and treatment that they need.

4. Parents and families cause eating disorders.

In the past, parents and families have been blamed for somehow "causing their children to develop eating disorders." For instance, there were theories that suggested that anorexia was caused by an overcontrolling mother. However, this idea that parents are somehow to blame for their child developing an eating disorder is utterly false.

Parents and families do not cause eating disorders. In addition, they can be incredible allies and sources of support for their loved ones in recovery.

5. There are only two types of eating disorders, anorexia and bulimia, or the other eating disorders are "less serious."

There are a variety of eating disorders that people suffer from. However, unfortunately media and public attention is primarily drawn only toward anorexia and bulimia.

While it is important to highlight the dangers of these illnesses, it's also crucial to recognize that binge eating disorder (BED) and otherwise specified feeding and eating disorder are just as serious and can also be life threatening.

Binge eating disorder is actually the most common eating disorder, but, unfortunately, it is often the least talked about. In addition, BED can have serious physical health complications and can be life threatening (National Eating Disorders Association 2016).

6. Eating disorders are all about food and weight.

Eating disorder symptoms manifest often in a fixation or disordered relationship to food and one's body. However, while eating disorder treatment certainty entails helping people to heal their relationship to food and their body, effective treatment goes beyond that.

It's important to note that nutritional rehabilitation and weight restoration (if the individual is under his or her set-point weight) is the first line of approach when it comes to treatment, as it is not effective to simply be doing talk therapy with someone who has a malnourished brain.

Often eating disorder symptoms serve some kind of function for an individual. For instance, individuals might use eating disorder behaviors in an attempt to regulate their emotions, cope with past trauma, or feel a sense of "comfort" or "calm."

In my work with people with eating disorders, part of the treatment is to begin to explore with them what "needs" their eating disorder is currently meeting in their life. Together, we then will look at some more life-affirming ways that they can begin to get their needs met.

7. You can never fully recover from an eating disorder.

There is also a common misconception that an eating disorder is an illness that one must suffer from forever. This belief can cause individuals to feel hopeless when it comes to working on their recovery.

However, with access to treatment and support, full recovery from eating disorders is completely possible. People can recover from their eating disorders and go on to lead productive and meaningful lives.

The Bottom Line

Through education and debunking common myths about eating disorders, we can help individuals who are struggling to seek life-saving treatment and further a better public understanding of these illnesses.

It is crucial that individuals who reach out for help are taken seriously and treated with compassion and care. No one chooses to have an eating disorder; however, people can make the choice to take positive steps in their recovery. Full recovery is possible.

Reference

"Binge Eating Disorder: Overview and Statistics." 2016. National Eating Disorders Association. https://www.national eatingdisorders.org/binge-eating-disorder. Accessed on June 20, 2017.

Jennifer Rollin, MSW, LCSW-C, is an eating disorder therapist in private practice in Rockville, Maryland. Her articles on eating disorders and body image issues have been published in a variety of media, including the Huffington Post *and* Psychology Today. *Connect with Jennifer at www.jenniferrollin.com.*

Traditional and Complementary Treatments for Binge Eating Disorder (BED)
Anjali A. Sarkar

The flickering shadows from the television set fell on the low table. A large plate of spaghetti and meatballs, four hamburgers, a platter of French fries and onion rings, a large bowl of chicken noodle soup, and a container of double-fudge ice-cream crowded every square inch of the low table. Sammy, stooped, and half-hidden under the fleece quilt ate swiftly, choking from time to time in her haste. Her mind and mouth were locked in an uncontrolled race against the digital clock on the mantel. She had to finish the food before the movie was over. She must. She washed it all down with a liter of Coke as the credits rolled on the screen.

Sammy, Samantha Barriner, 21, is not an isolated case. The National Eating Disorders Association reports 3.5 percent women and 2 percent men have binge eating disorder (BED) at some point in their lives, based on a study on 9,282 Americans published in *Biological Psychiatry* in 2007. BED is more commonly seen in women in their late teens or early twenties (Hudson et al. 2007).

The symptoms of binge eating include the following:

1. A secretive nature about food: Remember, BED is not just about overeating; it's also about being embarrassed about the overeating behavior, which leads to eating secretly, eating while alone, and hiding away any evidence of having eaten.

2. Food hoarding: Binge eaters tend to hide their stash of food away from all prying eyes.

3. Lack of control: Binge eating is accompanied by a lack of control over when and how much food is consumed.

4. Discomfort after eating: Since binge eaters eat way past their levels of satiety, they feel considerable physical discomfort after binging on food.

5. Abnormal eating regimen: Binge eaters do not follow any predictable pattern in eating and may skip several meals or eat very little and at odd times.

6. Eating rituals: Binge eaters are also seen to adhere to curious food rituals where they eat only a certain kind of food item (e.g., dairy) or need to have the food arranged in a certain order.

7. No purging: Binge eaters do not attempt to eliminate food from their bodies through forced vomiting or laxatives or other medication.

8. Mood swings: Most people suffering from BED also suffer from depression, anger, boredom, and stress.

9. Although most binge eaters are overweight or obese, not all patients of BED are overweight.

The primary challenge in the treatment for BED is the denial and extremely low self-esteem of patients, who hide their condition even from close family members and friends. Once diagnosed, a combined strategy of psychotherapy, medication, nutritional counseling, and group and family therapy help patients develop a sense of control over their eating behaviors.

Lisdexamfetamine dimesylate (Vyvanse) was the first drug to be approved by the Food and Drug Administration to treat BED in January 2015. The oral drug is a central nervous system stimulant and is also prescribed for attention deficit hyperactive disorder. Studies show Vyvanse helps reduce the number of binge eating episodes. However, the side effects of Vyvanse can be debilitating and include dry mouth, trouble sleeping (insomnia), increased heart rate (tachycardia), increased anxiety, psychiatric disorders, heart attack, and stroke. Another drug often prescribed for BED is topiramate (Topamax). However, Topamax has the side effects of memory loss, tingling sensations, speech problems, and drowsiness.

Recent research reveals an alternative approach to treatment for BED: yoga. Researchers at Deakin University show that a 12-week yoga program including postures, breathing, relaxation, and meditation in one 60-minute class per week, supplemented by a daily 30-minute personal yoga practice, reduced the number of binge eating episodes, as reported by patients themselves, improved self-esteem, and promoted a more positive body image. The program also resulted in a statistically significant decrease in body mass index and waist and hip circumference (McIver, O'Halloran, and McGartland 2009).

How yoga alleviates binge eating is a potential area of research. However, teachers believe that yoga provides the skills of identifying both positive and negative feelings in the moment and developing a nonjudgmental attitude toward such feeling. This increased tolerance and self-compassion, together with enhanced body awareness brought about by physical activity, help suppress the triggers for episodes of binge eating.

Recommended yoga practices for persons with BED include *Surya Namaskars* (sun salutations), balancing poses like *Vrykshasana* (tree pose), *Virabhadrasana III* (warrior pose III), *Trikonasana* (triangle pose), simple back bends like *Bhujangasana* (cobra pose), *Urdhva Mukha Shvanasana* (upward dog pose), *Salabhasana* (locust pose), and *Dhanurasana* (bow pose) and breathing techniques like *Bhastrika Pranayama* (bellow breath).

Sun salutations are the yogic equivalent of a cardio-workout and help increase circulation and oxygenation of the blood. Balancing poses, although apparently static, involve the constant dynamic adjustment of multiple agonistic and antagonistic muscle groups that engross the mind completely and provide a sense of grounding and accomplishment. The more challenging backbends elevate the mood through specific neural activation and also increase the metabolic rate. The bellow breathing technique increases vitality, reduces stubborn abdominal fat, activates the enteric nervous system, and increases metabolism.

Yoga curbs the internal negative self-talk through the mindful practice of postures and breathing. Attending regular yoga classes, and the sense of community it organically fosters, prevents the feeling of isolation and separation. Moreover, yoga philosophy offers, through the study of the *yamas* and *niyamas* (universal ethical guidelines and observances), an emotional framework that helps patients regain a sense of balance and control, not only with respect to their eating behaviors but also in developing a holistic perspective of their lives.

Psychologists and psychotherapists understand that the relationship a binge eater has with food is complex. A binge eater substitutes food for emotional bonds. Escaping into the world of binge eating is a patient's abnormal strategy of coping with the world. Yoga alleviates this escape route by bringing awareness to the present. Yoga forges a relationship with the body and the mind. This increased self-awareness, brought about by developing a diligent and regular practice, raises self-esteem and prevents all actions that abuse the body and the mind, including binge eating.

References

Hudson, J. I., et al. 2007. "The Prevalence and Correlates of Eating Disorders in the National Comorbidity Survey Replication." *Biological Psychiatry*. 61(3): 348–358. doi:10.1016/j.biopsych.2006.03.040.

McIver, S., P. O'Halloran, and M. McGartland. 2009. "Yoga as a Treatment for Binge Eating Disorder: A Preliminary Study." *Complementary Therapies in Medicine.* 17: 196–202.

Anjali A. Sarkar is a scientist with MindSpec Inc., Virginia, and works on neurobehavioral disorders. She holds a PhD in molecular biology and a master's degree in physiology. Dr. Sarkar has worked in the field of neurodevelopmental disorders for over 10 years. She is also a certified yoga teacher.

Removing the Thin Ideal from Your Home
Sharon Schroeder

I don't remember much about the vacation we took later, but I do remember the day that we were shopping for bathing suits for an upcoming vacation. My grandmother was on the phone with one of her twin daughters, the thin one. The favorite one. "You should see Sharon, she looks great! I swear she is just skin and bones!" I stood in the dressing room and looked at myself in the mirror as she spoke. I was thin. My skin was pale. The skin under my eyes appeared thin, and dark bags were the most noticeable feature on my face. The backs of my bottom teeth had already begun to decay, although that was not obvious to anyone but myself. I didn't look great; I looked unwell. But that I was thin was venerated, while my obvious signs of poor health were overlooked. I was proud to be noticed as thin; the rest didn't matter much.

Two years earlier, my grandmother had refused to let me buy a bikini because I was "too fat" for it, and that same summer she put me on Weight Watchers, except it was her own version of Weight Watchers, a more restrictive version. I knew I wasn't a thin girl, but I was okay with that. I liked the way I looked in a bikini, and I wanted to get tan on my belly. We compromised on a Tankini, while my underweight sister who was three years younger got a bikini. But in this tiny store, after a year and a half of my purging most meals, my grandmother was rushing around, phone in one hand and a selection of bikinis for me to choose from in the other. I couldn't bring myself to wear one that year; I refused to buy a bathing suit at all. Despite the praise, and despite seeing myself as thin, I hated my own body now. I spent the summer hiding every inch of my skin from the sun, refusing to enjoy some of my favorite activities, in favor of reading somber novels under a sheet on the beach or the boat. It gave me a great excuse for my sickly pale skin at least.

Thin idealism has been noted as a potential contributing factor to the development of eating disorders since the 1980s (Garner et al. 1982). Almost 10 years before I was born, as my mother suffered with her own undiagnosed disordered eating, the role of thin idealization began to be explored in depth. By the time I was 10 years old, thin ideal internalization was recognized as a causal factor in the development of body image issues and eating disorders (Thompson and Stice 2001). Today there are large-scale movements that operate under the goal of using dissonance-based intervention to counter the thin idealization in society and in our homes.

We can practice creating dissonance between thin ideal and health in our own communities. We can do this in our homes, at school, and with our friends. When viewing a magazine with friends, stopping to analyze the dramatic hair and makeup of the models in the high-end ads, you could mention that up to 94 percent of models are underweight and briefly note the negative health impacts of being underweight. You don't have to dominate the conversation to introduce dissonance.

We can practice dissonance at home, when our parents, partners, and children are struggling with their own body image issues. Does your mother talk about going to the gym to lose weight? Perhaps you could ask her if she has ever considered changing her motivations. Maybe you could help her find a way to see going to the gym as a pursuit in gaining strength rather than meeting an image that coincides with the thin ideal. Does your son talk about pursuing a body that is based on thin idealization? You can do your best to introduce dissonance by presenting the costs of pursuing the thin ideal, while promoting healthy bodies.

Small things, like presenting art that features women and men of healthy weights, can influence how one views one's own body. In Western society we are inundated with images of men and women who have extremely low body fat. Low body fat in and of itself is a health risk, and those health risks should be just as well known as the health risks that can be attributed to obesity. When we work to present images of healthy women and men in visible locations, we are actively countering thin idealism. Thin idealism advertises unhealthy bodies, while healthy bodies are not made visible in our society.

The things that everyone can do, no matter what relationships they have in their life, are plentiful. Weight discussions come up in almost any scenario. From the texts traveling between school classrooms to the cubicles of the tall buildings downtown, weight is discussed. If your friend texts you and asks you if you noticed the weight gain of a classmate, you could tell your friend that you're uncomfortable with such scrutiny on weight but that you did notice and like the classmate's new shirt. If you're in the office and a coworker refuses a donut, loudly asserting his or her intentions to lose weight, you could state that you are happy your coworker is choosing to limit the intake of nutrient-limited foods but that you'd love to see him or her make these choices for health reasons rather than image reasons.

If you are lucky enough to be the person that a child turns to when he or she has needs or curiosities, you have the greatest responsibility. Your words will be what that child's inner voice says to him or her and not just during his or her childhood but well into adulthood as well. Do you speak about losing weight? Restricting your food? Do you moralize food choice? Do you speak about restricting your child's food choices or your child's weight gain? Your child will remember. And you are not a bad person. Unpacking the messages of thin idealization is not easy. My eating disorder voice has not been quiet about how uncomfortable it feels about me writing these words. But I know that I have to stop, analyze, and reformulate my thoughts, because my community depends on people like me and my child does as well.

References

Garner, D., et al. 1982. "The Eating Attitudes Test: Psychometric Features and Clinical Correlates." *Psychological Medicine.* 12(4): 871–878.

Thompson, J. Kevin, and Eric Stice. 2001. "Thin-Ideal Internalization: Mounting Evidence for a New Risk Factor for Body-Image Disturbance and Eating Pathology." *Current Directions in Psychological Science.* 10(5): 181–183.

Sharon Schroeder is a 26-year-old mother who is recovering from a decade-long battle with eating disorders. With introspection and professional guidance, she is unpacking the damage of thin idealism within herself.

Food for Thought
Ivanna Soto

Music blasts from the speakers of the car as my sister and I sing along on our way to school. It's the same as usual; I'm driving; she's controlling the radio. As we pause at a stoplight, she puts on a new song I'd never heard of, an alternative one that I quickly catch on to, and she laughs at me as I yodel along to the tune as best I can. As the second verse comes on, I fall silent. "I want blood, guts, and angel cake," the singer croons. "I'm gonna puke it anyways . . ."

My sister continues to sing, but I'm quiet for the rest of the drive.

Modern-day media and celebrities have always been guilty of romanticizing mental illnesses, particularly eating disorders. Magazines talk about fad diets, and models confess to losing weight by not eating or by abusing drugs. As a teen-ager growing up in the United States, I would have been hard-pressed to escape the idealization of a thin, waif-like body, or the conditioning to view unhealthy eating habits as a normal thing. Eating disorders are often used as casual comments in conversation or punchlines—groans of "I'm so full I'm gonna throw up" after eating large meals or plus-size T-shirts that read "I overcame anorexia." As someone struggling with an eating disorder for seven years, I was used to hearing and ignoring these things, but this was the first time I had heard bulimia mentioned in a song that way.

Bulimia nervosa has always been like anorexia's less attrac-tive, awkward sister. No one wants to hear about teenage girls huddled over toilets, forcing themselves to gag until their stom-achs are empty. Despite 1.5 percent of women and 0.5 percent of men falling victim to bulimia in their lives—a significantly greater number than the 0.9 percent of women and 0.3 percent of men who become anorexic—awareness of the symptoms and effects of bulimia is disturbingly low among adults and teenagers ("Overview and Statistics" 2017).

I developed bulimia my freshman year of high school after struggling with body image issues for most of my life. It started slowly: eating a bit more than I meant to and feeling nauseous and then throwing up a bit. I felt better, and the next time I felt like I overate, I did it again, once a month, twice a week, until suddenly it became regular after every meal. Unaware of the symptoms of bulimia, I didn't realize it was starting to become a habit, that I was beginning to eat meals with the expectation of purging afterward. It wasn't until one day before a volleyball game, when I lied to my teammates about losing my phone so I could sneak off to the bathroom, that I realized this "one-time thing" had become an obsession.

Find the most private bathrooms in my area. Eat by myself. Find ways to sneak off to the bathroom alone. Joke about how much I eat to hide my binging habits. Take an aisle seat on an airplane so I don't bother people when I leave to lock myself in the tiny stall. I had developed habits that seemed unobtrusive to an unknowing eye, but that dominated my time and energy. And I was exhausted.

My mother and sister discovered my illness after a year of hiding it, and suddenly it became a new, even more draining game. They watched me with eagle eyes at every meal, and if I asked for seconds, I would get a snappish response: "So you can throw it up later? We can't afford to waste food!"

I felt horrible guilt and shame, knowing how much trouble I caused for everyone yet feeling powerless to stop. My sister was distrusting and almost cruel in her worry, constantly bringing up my bulimia in petty arguments. My mom was terrified. She pulled up page after page of horror stories: the girl with cancer in her throat, the boy with an ulcer in his stomach. She hoped one of them would snap me into awareness of what I was doing to my body and I'd make a decision to "cure myself." What she didn't realize is that I already knew. I knew my hair was thinning and my muscles were deteriorating. I knew I was wearing away at my teeth and throat, that the chemicals in my brain were becoming more and more unbalanced. When my mother, sobbing, shoved her phone in my face to show me an article about a girl who died from gastric rupture after a binge episode, I was completely unshaken. My only thought as I stared at the picture of the girl's bruised and distorted naked body hunched over a toilet was, I wonder when that will be me?

How many teens and young adults suffering from bulimia feel the same guilt and resigned dread that I did—and sometimes still do? Having to deal with my family's fear on top of my own made me realize how poorly eating disorders are dealt with, both among the victims and among their loved ones.

Eventually I was able to begin the journey to recovery, but it was not easy. It still isn't. Three years have passed since I tried to recover, and I still find myself relapsing. Each time I do, I think back on all the pain it's caused my family and me. Food is a part of staying alive, and when interacting with it becomes destructive, it's nearly impossible to escape. Overcoming an eating disorder is already challenging as it is, but once you add on the pressures of society and a poor support system, it can feel completely hopeless.

It took years for me to look past society's portrayals of eating disorders and my own family's behavior. I managed to find strength in a support system from my friends and a therapist, but I wonder if I could have avoided the pain I went through if there were better awareness about preventing and dealing with eating disorders. As we become more conscious of mental illnesses and how to fight them, I can only hope that parents and children alike are taught to better understand eating disorders, so they can help one another through such a struggle.

Reference

"Overview and Statistics." 2017. National Eating Disorders Association. https://www.nationaleatingdisorders.org/bulimia-nervosa. Accessed on May 30, 2017.

Ivanna Soto is an undergraduate at Yale University.

Eating Disorders in Adolescent Males
Jeremy Summers

For many teens, the pressure to subscribe to a singular notion of beauty can be overwhelming. This pressure leads to serious problems, such as low self-confidence, distorted self-image, and depression. Among the most serious of the problems caused by this type of pressure are eating disorders, which are classified as a variety of psychological disorders that are related by the prevalence of abnormal or disturbed eating habits. Eating disorders can wreak havoc on the still-developing organs of teens and can even be fatal, as organs can shut down from lack of proper nutrition. For generations, teenage girls have been at risk for developing eating disorders. In today's world, though, teenage boys are becoming increasingly at risk for developing eating disorders. In the United States alone, 20 million women and 10 million men will suffer from an eating disorder at some point in their life (Wade, Keski-Rahkonen, and Hudson 2011). While it is a challenge to find reliable data, it is clear that boys are burdened by the same pressures that were once felt by mostly girls and that gender can play a large role in the development of eating disorders.

Just a decade ago, the world was a very different place for teens. There was a fairly narrow range of acceptable behavior for both boys and girls, and straying outside of this range resulted in ridicule or worse. Now, though, evolving gender identities and definitions are blurring the traditional lines of what men and women should be. As a result, teenage boys have an added layer of confusion and difficulty when navigating their teenage years and have increased or greater expectations of being considered attractive and admired by their peers.

Unfortunately, when young men and women are faced with this sort of unrelenting pressure, they are susceptible to developing eating disorders. The three eating disorders affecting the greatest number of teens by percentage are anorexia nervosa (AN), categorized by an obsession with weight that leads to inadequate food intake, bulimia nervosa (BN), categorized by frequent episodes of eating large amounts of food followed by self-induced vomiting, and binge eating disorder (BED), categorized by frequent episodes of consuming large quantities of food but without self-induced vomiting, leading to extreme fluctuation in weight.

Though this area of research is still young, data prove that young boys are developing eating disorders at an alarming rate. In one of the most widely quoted studies in this area, males were found to have a lifetime prevalence of 0.3 percent for AN, 0.5 percent for BN, and 2 percent for BED (Hudson et al. 2007). But the pressure doesn't stop in high school. A 2013 study, which tested 1,383 adolescent males, found that prevalence of any clinically recognized eating disorder was 1.2 percent at age 14, 2.6 percent at age 17, and 2.9 percent at age 20

(Allen et al. 2013). This means that males are actually more susceptible as they grow out of their teenage years and into young adulthood. A 2011 study, involving 2,822 students at a large university, found that 3.6 percent of males had indicators of an eating disorder. The female-to-male ratio was 3:1 (Eisenberg et al. 2011).

One likely reason for the growing number of males with eating disorders is the evolving image of what a man should be. According to a study, most males want to be lean and muscular, which they think is the ideal male body type (Labre 2005). This has changed rather significantly since the 1970s, when a man could comfortably have a fuller physique and not be ridiculed for it.

In addition, many young males are desperate to increase their muscles. Nearly 25 percent of males in a normal-weight range think of themselves as underweight, while 68 percent of college-aged men think they have too little muscle ("Body-Image Pressure Increasingly Affects Boys" 2014). A staggering 90 percent of teenage boys have exercised in order to try to increase their muscle mass (Eisenberg 2011.

The pressure for young males to look like the actors they see in film and television is just as powerful as it is for young girls to do the same. In fact, it can be worse for young males, since they are often shamed when they admit they have a problem or seek treatment for it. It has been shown that the risk of mortality for males with eating disorders is actually higher than it is for females (Raevuori, Keski-Rahkonen, and Hoek 2014). In addition, men who suffer from eating disorders often suffer from other conditions, such as depression, substance abuse, and anxiety. Even when males do not suffer from clinically recognized disorders, they are still affected. Eating disorders not recognized at the clinical label, including binge eating, purging, and fasting, are nearly as common among males as females (Weltzin et al. 2014).

One of the biggest challenges to reliable statistics is the gender bias associated with assessment tests that have been used to identify eating disorders. Eating disorders have long been thought of as a problem exclusive to women, and men have been stigmatized if they are identified as having one of these disorders. While the stereotype of someone with an eating disorder might be a rich, white, adolescent girl, the truth is that eating disorders affect men and women, regardless of age or race. A recent study found that more than 99 percent of the books on eating disorders have a female bias (Cohn and Lemberg 2017).

Despite societal progress and increasing acceptance for nonconformity to traditional gender roles, men are still stigmatized and made to feel less manly if they seek treatment for an eating disorder. While additional research is certainly needed, it is clear that a growing number of men are struggling with eating disorders, and the medical community, as well as society at large, must continue to adjust their way of thinking when it comes to gender and eating disorders. Only when this stigma is removed will men and women alike have access to better, more effective treatment.

References

Allen, K., et al. 2013. "DSM-IV-TR and DSM5 Eating Disorders in Adolescents: Prevalence, Stability, and Psychosocial Correlates in a Population-Based Sample of Male and Female Adolescents." *Journal of Abnormal Psychology*. 122: 720–732.

"Body-Image Pressure Increasingly Affects Boys." 2014. *Atlantic*. https://www.theatlantic.com/health/archive/2014/03/body-image-pressure-increasingly-affects-boys/283897/. Accessed on May 15, 2017.

Cohn, Leigh, and Raymond Lemberg, eds. 2014. *Current Findings on Males with Eating Disorders*. London: Routledge.

Eisenberg, D., et al. 2011. "Eating Disorders Symptoms among College Students: Prevalence, Persistence,

Correlates, and Treatment-Seeking." *Journal of American College Health*. 59(8): 700–707.

Feldman, M., and I. Meyer. 2007. "Eating Disorders in Diverse, Lesbian, Gay, and Bisexual Populations." *International Journal of Eating Disorders*. 40(3): 218–226.

Hudson, J., et al. 2007. "The Prevalence and Correlates of Eating Disorders in the National Comorbidity Survey Replication." *Biological Psychiatry*. 61: 348–358.

Labre, M. 2005. "Burn Fat, Build Muscle: A Content Analysis of Men's Health and Men's Fitness." *International Journal of Men's Health*. 4(2): 187–200.

Raevuori, Anu, Anna Keski-Rahkonen, and Hans W. Hoek. 2014. "A Review of Eating Disorders in Males." *Current Opinions on Psychiatry*. 27(6): 426–430.

Wade, T. D., A. Keski-Rahkonen, and J. Hudson. 2011. "Epidemiology of Eating Disorders." In M. Tsuang and M. Tohen, eds. *Textbook in Psychiatric Epidemiology*, 3rd ed. New York: Wiley, 343–360.

Weltzin, T., et al. 2014. "Treatment Issues and Outcomes for Males with Eating Disorders." In Leigh Cohn and Raymond Lemberg, eds. 2014. *Current Findings on Males with Eating Disorders*. London: Routledge.

Jeremy Summers is a freelance science writer whose work has appeared in Forbes, RealClearScience.com, *and Truth about Trade .com, among others. He lives and works in North Carolina and is a graduate of Appalachian State University.*

The Gay Adonis Complex: Muscle Dysmorphia in Male Homosexuals
Michael Vallario

Muscle dysmorphia (MD) is defined as an obsessive preoccupation with one's own body in which there is a delusional or exaggerated belief that one's physique is too thin, too skinny, or not muscular enough. In many of these cases, the individual's body is either normal or even exceptionally muscular in spite of the preoccupation. The *Diagnostic and Statistical Manual of Mental Disorders—Fifth Edition* categorizes MD as a specifier for body dysmorphic disorder (BDD), in which there is an obsessive preoccupation with a certain aspect of an individual's appearance as being severely flawed and requiring efforts to mask or correct it (American Psychiatric Association 2013). MD is of particular concern with regard to gay men, who are already more susceptible to eating disorders than the general population (Kaminski et al. 2005). In addition, gay men tend to be especially preoccupied with muscularity even compared to heterosexual men (Chaney 2008). There exist a multitude of possible contributing factors accounting for the higher incidence of MD among gay men, including (but not limited to) social pressures within the gay community and at large, media influences, heteronormative and homonegative stressors, and psychological trauma.

MD and BDD may resemble eating disorders in several ways. In addition to general preoccupation with one's body, MD typically presents with a number accompanying behaviors, such as attempts at hiding or downplaying perceived defects, abnormal eating patterns, and excessive physical exercise (Pope et al. 1997). However, the distinction between MD and, for example, anorexia nervosa is that the preoccupations with size are inverted: since the goal is to always increase one's size, exercise is the primary focus, with dieting a secondary concern; the opposite is true in anorexia. The type of dieting often seen in those with MD includes meticulous monitoring of caloric intake, increased cardiovascular activity, and use of a variety of nutritional supplements, which, when performed in a prolonged manner, may also resemble pathological behavior (Probert and Leberman 2009). Individuals involved in competitions may incorporate controlled fasts, intentional dehydration, and use of diuretics to lower one's body fat percentage as much as possible without losing muscle mass. Years of adhering to such an austere lifestyle can cause immense psychological strain and obsessiveness around food intake and can also increase one's likelihood of developing a clinically recognized eating disorder. Consequently, the comorbidity between MD and eating disorders is two-fold: first, there are certain personality traits and psychological characteristics that can lead an individual to develop an eating disorder, MD, or both; second, once symptoms of MD are present, the individual is at a greater risk for developing an eating disorder due to the strict demands that usually coincide with preoccupation with muscular development.

There are a variety of proposed factors that impact the higher prevalence of MD among gay men. First, gay men as members of the sexual minority community represent a historically and pervasively subjugated minority group, with certain parts of the world still outlawing homosexuality completely, to the point that it is punishable by death (Shortnacy 2004). In addition, gay men may feel pressured to "achieve their masculine body images" in order to "compensate for the social perception of gay men as effeminate" (Eguchi 2011). Thus, one component behind the gay male drive for muscularity is the inherent lack of "maleness" associated and stereotyped with male homosexuality, which may result in attempts to counterbalance perceived effeminacy by building a large, muscular, powerful-looking frame. Chaney (2008) explains that the media may also be directly responsible for the increase in muscle dissatisfaction among men, in general, and that both mainstream and gay-specific fashion and exercise magazines influence perceptions on the type of physique that is held in highest esteem by society. Because of long-standing discrimination against nonheterosexual individuals and the minority stress that any oppressed group is vulnerable to, gay men are considered at risk for various forms of substance use, including anabolic steroids. Furthermore, many gay men who use anabolic steroids are also HIV positive, a relationship that began in the 1990s by physicians who prescribed them for HIV patients with wasting syndrome or myopathy (Berger et al. 1996). For some, MD is the culmination of decades of bullying or social rejection: teasing and ostracism during formative years can result in negative body attitudes in adulthood. All of the aforementioned factors that may be at the root of MD in one way or another can occur singularly or in combination with one another.

Overall, the psychological and miscellaneous ramifications for gay men with MD have been well documented and empirically supported. While there remain substantial ambiguity and overlap regarding which symptoms occur earliest or serve as predictors for MD, as opposed to those symptoms that develop as a result of MD, the clinical significance of all related issues should not be understated. Further research and investigation into more of the etiology of MD should be conducted, as well as specific endeavors to elucidate how sexual identity can complicate MD symptom presentation and severity. Most of the extant literature on MD acknowledges that there is also limited examination of how to help treat MD, as there are "no randomized controlled trials, and opinions are based on anecdotes and case reports" (Tod, Edwards, and Cranswick 2016). Perhaps once MD is better understood in all its complexity and diagnostic features, more adequate treatment interventions will be recommended to target it.

References

American Psychiatric Association. 2013. *Diagnostic and Statistical Manual of Mental Disorders*, 5th ed. Washington, DC: American Psychiatric Association.

Berger, J. R., et al. 1996. "Oxandrolone in AIDS-Wasting Myopathy." *Aids*. 10(14): 1657–1662.

Chaney, M. P. 2008. "Muscle Dysmorphia, Self-Esteem, and Loneliness among Gay and Bisexual Men." *International Journal of Men's Health*. 7(2): 157–170.

Eguchi, S. 2011. "Negotiating Sissyphobia: A Critical/ Interpretive Analysis of One 'Femme' Gay Asian Body in the Heteronormative World." *The Journal of Men's Studies.* 19(1): 37–56.

Kaminski, P. L., et al. 2005. "Body Image, Eating Behaviors, and Attitudes toward Exercise among Gay and Straight Men." *Eating Behaviors.* 6(3): 179–187.

Pope, H. G., et al. 1997. "Muscle Dysmorphia: An Underrecognized Form of Body Dysmorphic Disorder." *Psychosomatics.* 38(6): 548–557.

Probert, A., and S. Leberman. 2009. "The Value of the Dark Side: An Insight into the Risks and Benefits of Engaging in Health-Compromising Practices from the Perspective of Competitive Bodybuilders." *European Sport Management Quarterly.* 9(4): 353–373.

Shortnacy, M. B. 2004. "Sexual Minorities, Criminal Justice, and the Death Penalty." *Fordham Urban Law Journal.* 32(2): 231–236.

Tod, D., C. Edwards, and I. Cranswick. 2016. "Muscle Dysmorphia: Current Insights." *Psychology Research and Behavior Management.* 9: 179–188.

Michael Vallario is a clinical psychology, PsyD, student at Nova Southeastern University in Fort Lauderdale, Florida. He is enrolled in the Multicultural/Diversity track, which is his main area of interest. Michael completed clinical practica at an adolescent drug abuse prevention program and at a community mental health facility. He will be joining the interdisciplinary team at the Miami VA Spinal Cord Disorders and Injury Unit for elective practicum.

Real Boys Don't: A Recovering Anorexic's Perspective on Eating Disorders
Chris White

A recent report in the *Journal of Biological Psychiatry* indicates that at least 30 million Americans have suffered from an eating disorder at least once in their lifetime (Hudson et al. 2007).

Given the most recent estimate of the U.S. population accounts for some 321.4 million, that figure represents well over 10 percent, an estimate that does not take into account unreported or untreated cases. With a mortality rate of 5 percent per decade for anorexia nervosa alone (Smink, van Hoeken, and Hoek 2012), it is perhaps not unfair to state that it's difficult to overestimate the direct impact eating disorders play on millions of Americans' lives each day. Nor are eating disorders isolated occurrences. Recent studies have indicated that 50 percent of anorexia sufferers interviewed also reported diagnoses of clinical depression and mood disorder (Ulfvebrand et al. 2015). And much like other comorbid diseases, it's as difficult to distinguish a singular root cause as it is to treat it in a healthy and noncondescending fashion, difficult but not impossible.

Over the past few years, there has been a significant focus—and one demanding even greater examination—on the detrimental effects of unrealistic body images facing adolescent and postadolescent women. While the stigma that once revolved around eating disorders has not been entirely vanquished, more Americans are learning to engage in an open dialogue that addresses the epidemic with greater honesty and empathy. Indeed, the very appellate of "fat shaming" has become such a part and parcel of our everyday lexicon that it's hard to imagine a time in which healthier and accepting attitudes toward the natural diversity of body types didn't hold prevalence. As an adolescent growing up in the late 1980s and early 1990s, such an attitude would have been unthinkable. If eating disorders were examined, it was typically confined to made-for-TV movies and tabloid fodder and always with a hushed undertone of shame and secrecy. It was always someone else's problem, never imaginable to be thought of as occurring to your next-door neighbor and certainly never to either yourself or your family.

Stigma. It's the first step toward depersonalization. What better way to diminish the value of someone than by holding them to the standards of physical appearance, no matter how arbitrary or unnatural they might be? It's what a competitive society thrives on, isn't it?

I have no idea why I chose to starve myself for the first time as a 14 year old. Certainly there were mitigating factors. A recent diagnosis of low-level manic depression surely could have been one. A burgeoning—and altogether classically adolescent—disgust in both myself and my peers could also have contributed greatly. Even the deeply rooted guilt of being a bookish, slight and undeniably awkward teenager was bound to play some role in denying myself what was a basic necessity. In the end, you could likely say it was a penance for all three, plus a host of other nascent factors that took a good 25 years of my life to confront with any reasonable shred of dignity. But certainly, it was never a question of my masculinity. After all, real boys don't do those sort of things.

I'd be lying if I didn't say that the feeling of self-punishment was addictive—albeit in a highly dysfunctional way. Unlike drugs or drinking, the addiction felt like more of a conscious choice. I could have quit at any time and walked away with my masculinity intact because real boys don't do those sort of things.

By the time I was 17, I weighed approximately 95 pounds; and while I had never been in the least bit heavyset, the result of my physical appearance was enough to shock the most jaded eye. I learned to take pride in my skeletal features: my visible ribcage, my hollow, glassy eyes, and the veins peaking through my sallow arms like a road map. Pride in being grotesque, in being distorted, in appearing to be less than human. It was a quality that was uniquely my own: a mark of identity, one that no one could strip me of. But even this defective vanity came with a price. I had to learn to question my own identity as a man precisely because real boys don't do those sort of things.

Both my mother and teachers kept quiet. They suspected my appearance was the result of heavy drug use—which wasn't too far off. Like most teenagers, I learned to experiment with drugs and alcohol and, in my own case, developed a definite taste for both, which, for an adolescent who learned not only to survive but also to cherish the feeling of three square meals a week, is a recipe for disaster. When I was found unconscious at the bottom of a stairwell outside of a major highway overpass in Boston after three beers and hospitalized with what was most definitely a concussion, I was faced with two choices: a prolonged stay at a psychiatric and substance abuse clinic or continuing a toxic cycle and face an imminent early death. I chose the latter.

It wasn't until my second hospitalization that something snapped for me. There was something, some nagging little realization drilling itself into my head that made me realize that even despite my insecurities, my self-denial, my self-destruction, and a host of other malicious factors seeming to ooze out of every pore in my body, it came down to a choice: that it wasn't merely a question of failing to live up to standards of masculinity that were in no ways applicable to all walks of life, or letting teenage ennui swell up like some monstrous balloon, but a question of self-empathy. Not exactly the sensation of "rock bottom" so often alluded to in 12-step programs but not too distant either. The realization that self-respect and self-forgiveness aren't inherent but actively need to be worked for is foreign to many ways of thinking but then, again, so is anorexia.

The rationale behind eating disorders cannot be—and, in my opinion, should not be—systemized down to a handful of causes applicable to all. Because the human experience is so remarkably diverse—as diverse as body types, frankly—our experience of disorders is bound to be equally so. In fact, more so. Peer pressure, media distortion, self-loathing, or a cry for attention—these are all valid factors and ones that enjoy a much wider representation in the experience of eating disorders. But trying to slip a "one-size-fits-all" label onto any form of disorder does nothing to eliminate both its cause and effect. It is precisely because of our diversity that real men and real women feel pain. Real men and women cope in incredibly unhealthy ways. Real men and women abuse themselves. Real men and women crack under pressure. Real men and women cry real tears, real men and women feel very real pangs of fear and self-destruction, real men and women poison their bodies, real men and women learn to hate themselves, real men and women make very real choices, and ultimately real men and women die. But with the exception of the latter, real men and real women also recover.

References

Hudson, J. I., et al. 2007. "The Prevalence and Correlates of Eating Disorders in the National Comorbidity Survey Replication." *Biological Psychiatry*. 61(3): 348–358.

Smink, F. E., D. van Hoeken, and H. W. Hoek. 2012. "Epidemiology of Eating Disorders: Incidence, Prevalence and Mortality Rates." *Current Psychiatry Reports*. 14(4): 406–414.

Ulfvebrand, S., et al. 2015. "Psychiatric Comorbidity in Women and Men with Eating Disorders Results from a Large Clinical Database." *Psychiatry Research*. 230(2): 294–299.

Chris White is a writer and artist living in the Greater Boston area. His work has been published in periodicals, blogs, and anthologies, including several full-length novels under numerous pen names.

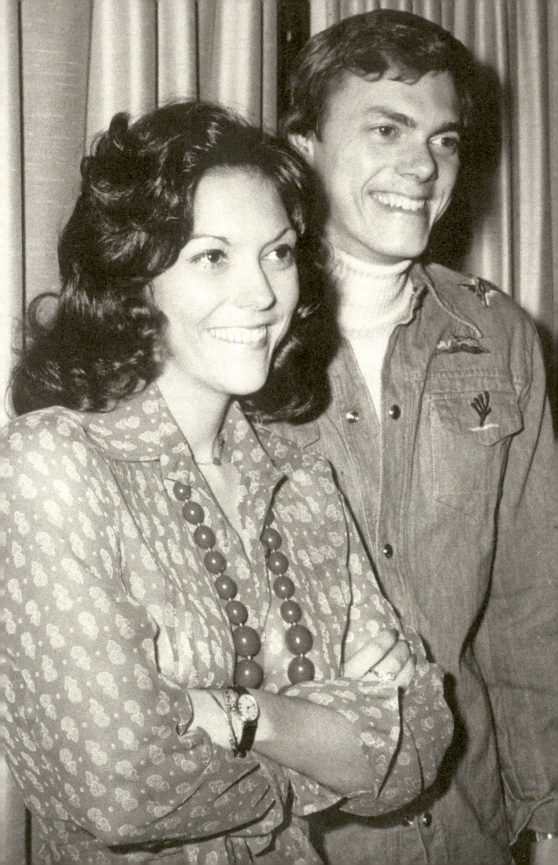

Introduction

The study of eating disorders is an inherent and profound human activity. The study of boys and girls and women and men, whose non-normal eating habits are a disruptive factor in their everyday lives, asks some of the basic questions one can imagine about human behavior. The search for ways to prevent and treat eating disorders similarly is an attempt to alter the most fundamental of all human behaviors: eating patterns. This chapter introduces some of the individuals and organizations that have been involved in this line of research, not only at the present time but also throughout history. The list of names included here is, and must be, limited by its very nature. But it provides an overview of the type of research and clinical work that is being and has long been done.

Academy for Eating Disorders

The Academy for Eating Disorders (AED) was founded on September 11, 1993, at a meeting held in Tulsa, Oklahoma, attended by 33 clinicians and researchers working in the field of eating disorders. Attendees shared a common concern about and commitment to improved treatment of and advocacy for individuals dealing with eating disorders, along with an

---

American pop duo Richard Carpenter and Karen Carpenter, backstage during a British tour in 1974. Karen Carpenter died from heart failure at the age of 32, as a result of her struggle with anorexia. (Keystone/Getty Images)

expanded and improved program of training for professionals in the field. By 2017, the organization had grown to a membership of more than 1,500 professionals in the field from more than 50 countries worldwide. Much of AED's work is carried out through special-interest groups, such as bariatric surgery; body image and prevention; child and adolescent eating disorders; dialectical behavior therapy; eating and sleep; epidemiology and public health practice; family-based treatment; genes and environment; health at every size; technology and innovations; lesbian, gay, bisexual, and transgender; males and eating disorders; medical care; neuroimaging; neuropsychology; new investigators; nutrition; professionals and recovery; psychodynamic and integrated psychotherapies; residential and inpatient; somatic and somatically oriented therapies; sport and exercise; student; substance use disorders; suicide; transcultural; trauma and eating disorders; and universities.

AED continues its tradition of a three-pronged emphasis: education, training, and research. Its website provides useful information, for example, on basic topics in the field of eating disorders, such as descriptions of all major eating disorders and treatment options. The organization also schedules regular webinars, twitter chats, and exchanges on various social media sites. Reference information on training in the field is also available for undergraduates and postdoctoral students via its student membership options, which also include access to special-interest groups for students. The AED website also contains a particularly useful and comprehensive list of reading resources on important topics in the field.

AED's research mission is carried by way of links to eating disorder research being carried out by institutions around the world. As of late 2018, for example, the AED website provided links to ongoing research studies at the University Health Network in Toronto, World Health Organization, Children's Hospital of Eastern Ontario, Helfgott Research Institute at National University of Natural Medicine Research Study, University of Miami Research Study on the Treatment of Adolescent

Eating Disorder Patients, UCLA Research Study on Anorexia Nervosa, La Trobe University Online Research Study, Stanford University Family-Based Treatment for Adolescent Anorexia Nervosa Research Study and Training, and Curtin University of Western Australia. The website also contains information about funding and training opportunities available in the field of eating disorders.

In addition to the organization's official journal, the *International Journal of Eating Disorders*, it provides a monthly newsletter, called *The Forum*, and a pair of guidelines publications, *Research Guidelines* (available in English, French, German, Italian, and Spanish) and the *Medical Care Standards Guide* (available in English, Chinese, French, and Brazilian Portuguese).

The Alliance for Eating Disorders Awareness

The Alliance for Eating Disorders Awareness (AEDA) is an organization based in West Palm Beach, Florida, that was founded in October 2000 with the goal of increasing public awareness of eating disorders and providing early intervention for men and women dealing with the disorder. It works to remove the secrecy and stigma associated with eating disorders and to provide a bridge between knowledge of the disorder and treatment services for those who are dealing with anorexia, bulimia, and other eating disorders.

AEDA claims to have provided support for more than 290,000 individuals in Florida, throughout the United States, and around the world in its nearly two decades of assistance, especially in improving self-esteem and a healthy body image for those dealing with an eating disorder. The organization was founded by Johanna Kandel after a personal long-term battle with eating disorders in her own life. Kandel now serves as CEO of the organization. She also published the story of her own life in her 2000 book, *Life beyond Your Eating Disorder* (Harlequin Nonfiction).

AEDA partners with a number of private facilities around the nation offering treatment services for eating disorders, including the ACUTE Center for Eating Disorders in Denver; Veritas Collaborative in Durham, North Carolina, Richmond, Virginia, and Atlanta, Georgia; Timberline Knolls, outside Chicago; and Viamar Health in West Palm Beach.

Alliance activities fall into four general categories: community education, professional training, "lunch and learn," and advocacy. The community education component involves a variety of programs dealing with eating disorders, with presentations on topics such as "Life beyond Your Eating Disorder"; "Debunking the Archaic Myth: Once You Have an Eating Disorder, You Will Always Have an Eating Disorder"; "Stepping Off the Scales: Eating Disorders and Body Image on College Campuses Inside"; "Eating Disorders: Struggles and Recovery"; "Eating Disorders and Males: It's Not Just a Girl Thing"; "Eating Disorders: When Exercise Is Not Always Healthy"; and "Promoting Positive Body Image in Children." Professional training services include programs for community educators, mental health practitioners, and health-care providers on topics such as Tools to Help Physicians/Nurses/Dentists Properly Screen, Assess, and Diagnose Eating Disorders; Dual Diagnosis: Eating Disorders and Substance Abuse; Eating Disorders and Abuse; Making Weight: Eating Disorders and Athletes; The Other Eating Disorders; and Eating Disorders and Personality Disorders. All programs are offered at no charge to participants.

Another free activity is the organization's "Lunch and Learn" program, which involves presentations for doctors, nurses, public health workers, and others who may come into contact with eating disorder problems. These programs offer information on the nature of eating disorders, screening criteria, and diagnostic techniques and procedures. The AEDA advocacy effort focuses on letter-writing to legislators and other decision makers, as well as regular lobbying visits to Washington, D.C., and state capitols, where information is presented on eating disorder issues.

A very useful service provided by the organization is the "Information" page of its website. This page provides basic information on a number of eating disorder–related issues, such as an explanation as to what eating disorders are; the types of eating disorders that have been identified; special information about eating disorders for boys and men; self-harming behaviors; the causes of eating disorders; debunking of myths about eating disorders; and specialized information for family and friends, educators, and coaches.

Binge Eating Disorder Association

The Binge Eating Disorder Association (BEDA) was founded in 2008 by Chevese Turner, a woman who has had a long history of the disorder. Her compelling online biography describes her earliest experiences with overeating even as a child and her eventual success as an adult in learning the nature of her problem and developing methods for dealing with it. Only after an ill-advised surgical procedure and consequent commitment to intensive therapy with a team of experts in eating disorders was she able to deal successfully with her eating issues. At that point, she understood that an important element of binge eating disorder is the lack of information about the condition, both among those who are dealing with binge eating and among the general public. She also became aware of the gap between knowing about the condition and finding dependable ways of dealing with the disorder. At that point, she decided to create an organization—BEDA—to deal with these two issues.

Its current mission statement explains that BEDA focuses on "providing leadership, recognition, prevention, and treatment of BED and associated weight stigma. Through outreach, education and advocacy, BEDA facilitates increased awareness, proper diagnosis, and treatment of BED." BEDA's statement of values provides an even better insight into the specific objectives it hopes to achieve, such as

- providing understanding and hope about binge eating disorder;
- supporting evidence-based research;
- promoting clinically accepted practices;
- collaborating with organizations to create awareness of BEDA;
- educating clinicians about ways of providing equitable treatment; and
- advocating for BED awareness and weight stigma prevention at all levels of education, government, and policy.

One section of the BEDA website focuses on fundamental information about binge eating, such as causes of the disorder, risk factors for and causes of BEDA, possible complications of the disorder, treatment options, issues to deal with before and during treatment, and the recovery process. The organization's two main events of the year are its annual conference and its BEDA National Weight Stigma Awareness Week. The latter event is subtitled "Teaching Kids the Truth" and consists of daily podcasts, blog posts, videos, free downloadable posters, weight stigma toolkits, and a general overview of the annual conference.

In addition to a good collection of books, articles, and Internet resources on binge eating disorder, the association provides "toolkits" for providers and for individuals, families, and friends. The former provides information about weight stigma, how it may arise in one's professional practice (intentionally or not), and how it can be dealt with. Specific toolkits are available for nutrition counseling; fitness professionals, physical therapists, and massage therapists; psychotherapists; physicians and other health-care providers; and school programs. The second toolkit provides general information about binge eating disorder, along with suggestions for ways in which one can provide assistance and support for someone dealing with the condition. BEDA also acts in the political arena to educate decision makers about the nature of binge eating and ways in which the government can assist in dealing with the problem. It provides members and the general public with information about pending actions at the national and state levels that may impact those with eating disorder and recommends ways in which those individuals can influence such actions.

Hilde Bruch (1904–1984)

Bruch was one of the most important figures in the history of research on eating disorders. She devoted more than 40 years to the study of anorexia and obesity and the factors that contributed to their development. Her first book on the subject, *Eating Disorders: Obesity, Anorexia, and the Person Within*, published in 1973, reflected her approach to the subject, focusing on the individual with an eating disorder rather than on the disorder itself. Her later book, *The Golden Cage: The Enigma of Anorexia Nervosa* (1977), presented her research findings in a format designed for the lay reader, especially those individuals who were struggling with anorexia or obesity. The last book she wrote, *Conversations with Anorexics*, was completed only days before she died.

Hilde Bruch was born on March 11, 1904, in the German town of Dülken, near the Dutch border. Her family was active in the local Jewish community, although the town itself was predominantly Catholic. She was the third of seven children born to Hirsch and Adele (Rath) Bruch, who owned a livestock business in the largely rural community. Bruch later related the joys she experienced growing up in the lush countryside. She had modest expectations of her life as a child, later telling a biographer that her goal in life at an early age was to "become a mother."

For her primary education, Bruch attended a one-room Jewish school in Dülken, where she later wrote that she was "a very disturbing student, because I asked questions. I was very well behaved but I never believed a thing" ("Papers of Hilde Bruch"

1985). At the age of 10, she enrolled at the local high school but remained there for only two years. She left the school at the age of 12 because she had heard of another school in the nearby town of Gladbach where "girls could study whatever they wanted," an option that was not available in her hometown.

By the time Bruch graduated from high school in 1923, she had changed her career choice from "mother" to "mathematician." An uncle soon convinced her, however, that medicine would be a more suitable career for a Jewish woman, and that was the field of study she selected when she entered the Albert Ludwig University in Freiburg im Breisgau. After receiving her MD in 1929, Bruch accepted a research appointment at the University of Kiel for one year, following which she spent a second year at the University of Leipzig. At the conclusion of her research studies at Leipzig, she decided to open a private practice in the town of Ratingen, near Düsseldorf, Germany.

That period in German history was one of tumult and revolution, however. Germany was suffering from the worst economic crisis in memory. Burdened with a crushing debt imposed by the victors of World War I, the German government struggled to provide even the most basic level of living for its citizens. That condition led in 1934 to the election of Adolf Hitler as president of the German Republic. Almost immediately, the new ruling National Socialist (Nazi) party began to implement a number of repressive measures against minorities, most prominently Jews. Bruch understood very quickly that the new German government—and probably German citizens in general—were unlikely to be congenial to the presence of a Jewish doctor, male or female, in the new society. By April 1933, the German government had issued a number of edicts, specifically banning Jews from a number of (most) professions, including medicine and medical research. Bruch saw the "writing on the wall," and, overcoming trepidations about leaving her family in Germany, she accepted an appointment at London's East End Maternity Hospital. In 1934, she moved again, this time to New York City, where she took a position as an assistant in pediatrics at the Babies Hospital.

After only a year in New York, Bruch was hospitalized for severe depression, brought on largely by her worries about the fate of her family in Germany. The therapy she received during that time introduced her to the field of psychiatry, about which she had known relatively little. Concurrently, Bruch was assigned the care of some young children at the hospital, who were suffering from eating disorders. She assumed at first that the disorders were caused by an endocrinology problem but failed to prove that hypothesis. Instead, it finally became clear to her that the disorders were caused by familial factors, such as the care (or lack of it) provided by mothers for their babies. On the basis of her own treatment for depression and her studies of babies' eating disorders, Bruch decided to change the focus of her career and concentrate on the field of psychiatry. Thus, she left Babies Hospital in 1941 to begin her studies at the Children's Psychiatric Service of the Johns Hopkins Hospital and the Henry Phipps Psychiatric Clinic, while also doing her training in psychoanalysis at the Washington–Baltimore Psychoanalytic Institute. At the conclusion of her psychiatric training, Bruch returned to New York City, where she opened a private practice and assumed a teaching post at Columbia University College of Physicians aril Surgeons. She was eventually appointed to the post of full professor there in 1959.

In 1964, Bruch was invited to move to Houston, Texas, to become professor of psychiatry at the Baylor College of Medicine. She held that title until 1978, when she retired and was named professor emerita at Baylor. By that time, she was in the early stage of Parkinson's disease, a condition that would eventually completely disable her and, on December 15, 1984, lead to her death. Bruch was honored with a number of awards in her lifetime, including the President's Citation for Meritorious Contributions to the Clinical Services of Baylor College of Medicine (1978), William A. Schonfeld Award for Contribution to Psychiatry of the American Society for Adolescent

Psychiatry (1978), the Golden Doctoral Diploma of the Medical Faculty of Albert–Ludwig University of Freiburg (1978), the Mount Airy Gold Medal Award for Distinction and Excellence in Psychiatry (1979), the Nolan D. C. Lewis Award for Contributions to Psychiatry (1980), the American Psychiatric Association Founders Award (1981), the Agnes Purcel McGavin Award of the American Psychiatric Association (1981), and the Joseph B. Goldberger Award in Clinical Nutrition of the American Medical Association (1981).

Cynthia M. Bulik (1960–)

Bulik is one of the nation's and world's most distinguished researchers in the field of eating disorders. She has been studying and teaching and writing on the topic since 1982 and has developed inpatient, outpatient, and partial hospitalization treatment programs for eating disorders in the United States and New Zealand. She is the author of about 40 chapters in anthologies and more than 400 peer-reviewed papers on eating disorders. She has served as associate editor of the *International Journal of Eating Disorders*, consulting editor of the *Journal of Abnormal Psychology*, and reviewer for more than 50 professional journals. She has also been the recipient of more than 75 grants and awards for the conduct of her research.

Cynthia Marie Bulik was born on February 13, 1960, in Pittsburgh, Pennsylvania. She studied at the Interpreters' Institute at the University of Salzburg from 1977 through 1978 and the University of Notre Dame, from 1978 through 1982, from which she received her BA in psychology and modern languages. She then continued her studies at the University of California at Berkeley, where she earned her MA in clinical psychology in 1985 and her PhD in the same field in 1988. She then completed two postdoctoral fellowships in the department of psychiatry at the University of Pittsburgh School of Medicine during 1988–1989 and 1989–1990.

Bulik's work experience includes positions in research, teaching, and clinical assignments. Among these assignments have been research assistant at Notre Dame; research fellow and research associate in psychiatry at the University of Pittsburgh; associate professor and professor at the Medical College of Virginia; professor of psychiatry and nutrition at the University of North Carolina; behavior therapist at the Anxiety Disorders Clinic of the University of Pittsburgh; senior clinical psychologist at the Eating Disorders Service of the Princess Margaret Hospital in Christchurch, New Zealand; director of the Eating Disorders Program at the Medical College of Virginia; and director of the Eating Disorders Program at the University of North Carolina, a position she continues to hold today. In addition to her academic work, Bulik served as figure skating coach for the Michiana Figure Skating Association from 1979 through 1982 and at the Richmond (Virginia) Ice Zone from 1999 through 2003. From 2010 through 2014, Bulik led the 18-nation Genetic Consortium for Anorexia Nervosa, of which she was founder. She was also one of the founders and leaders of the Anorexia Nervosa Genetics Initiative at the University of North Carolina, an effort to find genetic clues that may be associated with the disorder.

Bulik has received more than three dozen honors and awards during her career, including the Notre Dame Scholar Award (1978), Mellon Research Fellowship in Psychiatry (1980), Distinctive Achievement in Psychology Award (1982), Founder Region Soroptomists' Fellowship (1986), Phi Beta Kappa Dissertation Award (1987), Young Investigator Travel Award (1989), Richmond Magazine Top Doctors for Women: Eating Disorders (2001), R. O. Jones Memorial Lecture of the Canadian Psychiatric Association, President of the Academy for Eating Disorders (2003–2004), Eating Disorders Coalition Research Award (2004), Special Recognition for Support, Prevention and Work with Eating Disorders in Mexico of the Hispano Latino American SIG (2004), Hulka Innovators Award (2005), Carolina Women's Center Women's Advocacy Award

(2005), Academy for Eating Disorders Leadership in Research Award (2006), The Price Family National Eating Disorders Association Award for Excellence in Research (2008), Women's Leadership Council Faculty-to-Faculty Mentorship Award (2009), IAEDP Honorary Certified Eating Disorders Specialist (2009), František Faltus Award from the Czech Psychiatric Society of the J. E. Purkyne Czech Medical Society (2011), and the Meehan Hartley Advocacy Award of the Academy for Eating Disorders (2011).

Karen Carpenter (1950–1983)

It seems likely that no single individual in modern history has so focused public attention on the problem of eating disorders than did Karen Carpenter. A very successful popular singer, Carpenter died in 1983 from heart failure that developed as a result of her ongoing problem with anorexia nervosa.

Karen Anne Carpenter was born in New Haven, Connecticut, on March 2, 1950. Her parents were Harold Bertram Carpenter and Agnes Reuwer Tatum Carpenter. At the age of 13, Karen moved with her parents and her brother Richard to Downey, California, where she attended Downey High School. She joined the school band, where she at first was asked to play the glockenspiel. Not particularly enamored of the instrument, she asked to join the percussion section instead, where she soon became proficient on the drums. While still in high school, Karen and Richard formed their first band, with Richard on the piano, Karen on the drums, and a friend, Wes Jacobs, on the bass and tuba. The band entered a competition at the Hollywood Bowl in 1966, which they won, earning them a contract with RCA Records. Nothing came of the contract, however, as the company expressed its doubts about the likely success of a band that featured a jazz tuba. During the period, Richard and Karen made their first recordings in 1965 and 1966.

Karen's first experience with dieting came in 1967 in reaction to comments by friends that she was a bit "chubby."

To deal with these observations, she decided to try losing weight by going on the Stillman Diet, also known as the Quick Weight Loss Diet. The diet recommendations include lean meats, seafood, and eggs and exclude high-fat and high-carbohydrate foods. The diet plan recommends that one eat six small meals a day, instead of the traditional three larger meals, and includes consumption of at least eight glasses of water a day. The diet plan worked for Karen, whose weight dropped from 145 pounds before dieting to 120 pounds in the early 1970s to 91 pounds in 1975. She weighed 108 pounds at the time of her death. (Karen stood 5 feet 5 inches in height.) Cause of her death was determined to be emetine cardiotoxicity, secondary to anorexia nervosa. *Emetine cardiotoxicity* is a term used to describe a condition produced by the over-the-counter medication emetine (ipecac) on the heart. The most common use of ipecac is to induce vomiting, particularly in cases in which an individual has swallowed a poison. Presumably Carpenter was ingesting the medicine for reasons other than poisoning.

In their relatively brief career, the Carpenters achieved some of the highest awards in popular music. From 1970 through 1977, they were nominated for a number of Grammy Awards, including Best New Artist; Best New Artist Best Contemporary Vocal Performance by a Duo, Group or Chorus; Best Pop Vocal Performance by a Duo or Group; Song of the Year; Album of the Year; Record of the Year; Best Instrumental Arrangement; and Best Engineered Recording. They won the Grammy in the first three of these categories. Karen also received a number of awards and recognition for her own work, including *Playboy* magazine's Best Drummer of the Year in 1975, the number 29 ranking on the 100 Greatest Women of Rock and Roll in 1999, and number 94 on *Rolling Stone* magazine's 100 Greatest Singers of All Time. Carpenter's life story has been presented in a motion picture, *Superstar: The Karen Carpenter Story* (1987); a made-for-TV movie, *The Karen Carpenter Story* (1989); and two documentaries, *Close to You: Remembering the Carpenters* (1997) and *Only Yesterday: The Carpenters Story*

(2007). Karen's life and her struggles with anorexia have been memorialized in a number of books, including *Little Girl Blue: The Life of Karen Carpenter*, by Randy L. Schmidt and Dionne Warwick (2010); *The Carpenters: The Untold Story: An Authorized Biography*, by Ray Coleman (1994); *Karen Carpenter*, by Tom Stockdale (2000); and *Some Kind of Lonely Clown: The Music, Memory, and Melancholy Lives of Karen Carpenter*, by Joel Samberg (2015).

Caterina di Giacomo di Benincasa, Saint Catherine (1347–1380)

Catherine was one of the most famous of the so-called miraculous maids, who could be found in a number of countries in Western Europe from the Middle Ages to the end of the nineteenth century. A common characteristic of these women was that they greatly restricted their intake of food as a symbol of their commitment to the teachings of the Roman Catholic Church.

Catherine Benincasa was born in Siena, Italy, on March 25, 1347. At the time, the city and country were being ravaged by the Black Death, an epidemic that killed up to half the population of many areas in Europe. Catherine's mother was the daughter of a prominent local poet, and her father was a dyer of cloth. Her mother, Lapa, was extraordinarily fecund, producing a total of 25 children during her lifetime, half of whom died at, or shortly after, their birth. Catherine's own twin sister, Giovanna, survived only a few weeks after her birth.

Catherine began having religious and mystical experiences at a very early age. When she was about five, she is said to have had a vision of Christ seated with three of his apostles while walking home from a visit with her older sister Bonaventura. Her confessor later wrote that she was so impressed by this experience that she decided to "give her life to Christ" at the age of seven.

Another critical event occurred when Catherine was about 15. Bonaventura died in childbirth, and Lapa arranged for

Catherine to be married to Bonaventura's widowed husband. Having heard from her sister that her husband was a cruel man, Catherine entirely rejected the marriage plan. To reinforce her decision, she started fasting, a practice that she continued to follow for the rest of her life. On the advice of her confessor, Catherine attempted to take some food at least once every day. But she found that she was unable to hold the food down and vomited after every meal. She said that whether or not she might want to eat, God did not want her to do so, and he indicated this desire by forcing her to reject food.

By her late teens, Catherine had begun to devote her life entirely to prayer, contemplation, and care for the sick and homeless. Over time, she withdrew more into her own small cubicle at her parents' home, during which time she is said to have survived for months with no more than a sip of water each day and, in some cases, a bit of a communion wafer.

At the age of 16, Catherine had another vision, this time of St. Dominic, and interpreted the vision as a command to join the saint's convent at Mantellate. Her mother strongly opposed this idea and relented only when Catherine came down with a terrible rash, accompanied by a fever and severe pain. When her mother took this as a sign of God's will that Catherine be allowed to join the convent, she did so and was immediately cured of her illness. At the age of 21, Catherine experienced yet another vision, one in which she was joined in marriage to Jesus. Thereafter, she claimed to be his wife and proved the fact with the wedding ring she received at the marriage, which was, perhaps fortuitously, invisible.

During her years as a Dominican tertiary (a lay position below that of monks ["primaries"] and nuns ["secondaries"]), Catherine continue her practice of self-starvation. Over time, she became weaker and more prone to illness, and she eventually died, probably as a final consequence of the practice, in Rome on April 29, 1380.

During the few years of her life, Catherine became very active politically, in an effort to return the papacy from Avignon to Rome. She also made an effort to convince Gregory that reform of the church was essential, an effort in which she had no success. Among the miracles attributed to Catherine, in addition to the visions mentioned here, were her ability to elevate a few inches above ground during moments of adoration and meditation, the ability to go many weeks without sleeping, and the receipt of the stigmata (the appearance of a sword-caused cut in her side, in the same position as that received by Jesus on the cross). After her death, cures to the sick were credited to their visit to the saint's grave in Rome. Based on these many miracles, Catherine was canonized by Pope Pius II on June 29, 1461.

Eating Disorder Hope

Eating Disorder Hope (EDH) was founded in January 2005 by Jacquelyn Ekern, who herself recovered from an eating disorder. EDH is the "doing-business-as" name for Ekern Enterprises, Inc., which Jacquelyn and her husband operate out of Redmond, Oregon. The organization's overall philosophy is to promote the ending of "eating disordered behavior, embracing life and pursuing recovery." Its mission is to "foster an appreciation of one's uniqueness and value in the world, unrelated to appearance, achievement or applause."

The organization's website is a gold mine of information about all aspects of eating disorders, including specialized web pages on eating disorders, in general; eating disorder statistics; specific eating disorders, such as anorexia nervosa, bulimia nervosa, and binge eating disorder; weight and body image; excessive exercise, nutrition, and orthorexia; food addiction; dialectical behavioral therapy; cognitive behavioral therapy; nutrition therapy; family therapy; art therapy; dance and movement therapy; equine therapy; acceptance and commitment therapy; interpersonal psychotherapy; exposure and response prevention therapy; eating disorder support groups;

spirituality and eating disorders; teen, children, and adolescent eating disorders; eating disorders in men; middle-aged women and eating disorders; athletes and eating disorders; pregnancy and eating disorders; affording and paying for eating disorder treatment; compulsive spending and eating disorders; weight-loss surgery and eating disorders; dieting and eating disorders; diabetes and eating disorders; families and eating disorders; medical complications from eating disorders; dual diagnosis and co-occurring disorders; and family involvement in treatment.

As part of its overall mission, EDH has created special-interest groups for targeted individuals dealing with eating disorders. Currently, they include College Hope, for college students; Eating Disorder Hope for Professionals, designed for individuals who work in the field of eating disorders research, prevention, and treatment; and the Career Center for Eating Disorder Professionals, aimed at individuals who wish to pursue a career in the eating disorders profession. EDH's website also provides a superb interactive search engine for eating disorder treatment centers in all 50 states and the District of Columbia, along with similar online resources. The organization also provides a variety of support activities on its website, including a blog and vblog through which individuals can share their own experiences with eating disorders, along with a support forum in which one can obtain advice, guidance, and support in dealing with one's own unique eating issues.

Other support activities available on the EDH website include webinars and twitter chats, eating disorder recovery tips and self-help suggestions, inspirational stories about eating disorder recovery, and a discussion of the role of spirituality in dealing with eating disorders. The organization also provides links to books on various aspects of eating disorders. A very helpful and detailed calendar of coming eating disorder events is also available on the EDH website.

In January 2013, Ekern founded a sister organization to EDH, Addiction Hope. The organization was created because many people struggling with an eating disorder also have co-occurring addictions of various kinds. The primary fields of interest for Addiction Hope, in addition to eating disorders, are substance abuse, mental health, recovery and support, and treatment options. The organization's website is https://www .addictionhope.com/.

Eating Disorders Anonymous

Eating Disorders Anonymous is a fellowship of individuals who commit to the Alcoholics Anonymous (AA) model for recovery created in the 1930s by "Bill W" (William Griffith Wilson) to help alcoholics deal with their alcohol problems. The basis of the AA model is a set of 12 steps and 12 traditions to which a person commits. Both the 12 steps and the 12 traditions are deeply embedded in spiritual/religious traditions and philosophy, although AA and later organizations formed on the same model interpret these basic concepts in the most general way possible. The success of AA in aiding recovery from alcoholism later led to the development of similar programs for other life issues, such as Drug Addicts Anonymous, Cocaine Anonymous, Crystal Meth Anonymous, Marijuana Anonymous, Gamblers Anonymous, Overeaters Anonymous, Sexaholics Anonymous, and Debtors Anonymous. Similar groups, such as Al-Anon and Nar-Anon, have also been created to assist family and friends of addicts in dealing with their issues. Eating Disorders Anonymous (EDA) was founded in 2000 by a small group of AA members who discovered that they had similar issues and decided that the 12-step, 12-tradition model might be a mechanism for helping them to deal with the eating disorder issues.

As with other 12-step programs, EDA is structured rather loosely with no dues or formal organization. The only requirement is that one commit toward the goals and methods of the organization and toward regular attendance at EDA meetings. A typical EDA meeting involves a brief opening ceremony (reading of the 12 traditions), followed by a short biographical talk given by one of the members, and concluding with testimonies from individual members about their own history of eating disorders. A social hour often follows the meeting at which individuals can exchange personal stories and encouragement.

People who commit to EDA should understand that the organization does not provide any kind of formal program for dealing with eating disorders, as one might find in a traditional treatment center. It, for example, offers no specialized recommended eating program or any professional agenda for recovery from the addiction. Instead, members turn the solution of their problem over to a higher power for guidance as to how their own recovery is going to occur. In its own commentary on the organization's purpose, EDA says that, for members, "recovery means living without obsessing on food, weight and body image."

The EDA website provides links to individual groups located in 42 states, the District of Columbia, and 10 foreign countries. In addition, it provides a schedule of online meetings for individuals who are unable to locate or attend live meetings. As with other 12-step groups, EDA has written a special publication with information for its members, the *Big Book on Eating Disorders*. The book is available for purchase in hard cover and, at no cost, online at the EDA website. The organization also offers a variety of print and digital publications in the form of EDA Meeting Starter Kits, brochures on various specific topics ("Could You Be One of Us?" "Are You New to the 12 Steps or Sponsorship?" "Information for Professionals," "EDA at a Glance," "EDA Recovery, Milestones and Balance," "EDA Recovery Tools," "Service as a Solution," and "EDA on Binge Eating/Anorexia/Bulimia/OSFED/Emotional Eating"), and general publications on topics of interest to individuals with eating disorders. The organization also held its first (to be annual) "Big Book Study Workshop" for all members in July 2017, in Chicago.

Eating Disorders Coalition

The Eating Disorders Coalition for Research Policy and Action (usually known simply as the Eating Disorders Coalition [EDC]) was formed in 2000 for the purpose of promoting a better understanding of and more extensive action on eating disorder issues at the national, state, and local levels. Individuals can support the mission of the EDC in one of two ways, either by connecting with the organization online through social media groups such as Facebook, Instagram, Twitter, or Google+ or by joining the organization's mailing list, or by becoming a friend of the EDC by making a monetary contribution of $100 per year. As of late 2017, 10 individuals were listed as members, along with others who preferred to remain anonymous. In addition to individual members, a number of organizations are listed under one of seven "circles" of support: Hope, Support, Advocacy, Leadership, Policy, Executive, and Champions. Representative of each category are Gurze Books, Mothers against Eating Disorders, Center for Change, Remuda Ranch Treatment Center, the Renfrew Center, Kantor & Kantor, LLP, and National Eating Disorders Association, respectively.

As listed on its website, the goals of EDC are as follows:

- Raise awareness among policy makers and the public at large about the serious health risks posed by eating disorders
- Promote federal support for improved access to care
- Increase resources for education, prevention, and improved training
- Increase funding and support for scientific research on the etiology, prevention, and treatment of eating disorders
- Promote initiatives that support the healthy development of children

- Mobilize concerned citizens to advocate on behalf of people with eating disorders, their families, and professionals in the field

As of late 2017, the organization was focused on a handful of especially important issues: working to promote the rule-making process in connection with the Anna Westin Act and provisions of the 21st Century Cures Act dealing with eating disorders; ensuring a smooth transition that protects the rights of those with eating disorders from the Affordable Care Act (ACA) to whatever system replaces it; and lobbying for eating disorder provisions under the Peer Reviewed Medical Research Program. The organization has been acting in support of other legislative actions, such as Medicaid provisions of the House-passed 2017 Americans Health Care Act (AHCA), expansion of parity in mental health programs in the state of New York, the Preventative Health Savings Act, and the AspireAssist act that provides technology for the treatment of obesity.

Some of the organization's previous initiatives had involved advocacy for the Truth in Advertising Act of 2014; the Federal Response to Eliminate Eating Disorders Act of 2013; Eating Disorders Awareness, Prevention, and Education Act of 2000, 2001, 2003, 2005, and 2007; Promoting Healthy Eating Behaviors in Youth Act of 2002; and Improved Nutrition and Physical Activity Act of 2002, 2003, 2005, 2006, and 2007. Other previous policy initiatives had been directed at obtaining mental health parity for eating disorders, opposing BMI testing in schools, influencing the implementation of the ACA, increasing funding for eating disorders by the National Institutes of Health, challenging educational programs to reduce obesity, and requiring insurance companies to provide coverage for eating disorders.

In its summary of past achievements, EDC lists such accomplishments as working to improve existing bills dealing with eating disorders, introducing new bills on the condition, and being involved in the adoption of relevant bills at the federal and state levels. In addition, it has been successful in promoting research and educational programs on eating disorders at the U.S. Centers for Disease Control and Prevention and the Department of Health and Human Services.

The EDC website contains a page on Facts and Information, which provides basic information on eating disorders in general and specific conditions. It also has an especially useful collection of information on the meaning and implementation of mental health parity for eating disorders programs and the provisions in insurance policies for payment of eating disorder treatment. The section also contains a listing of current research programs dealing with one or another phase of eating disorders, some of which are searching for volunteer participants.

Elisa Project

The Elisa Project was founded in 1999 by Rick and Leslie McCall, in honor of their daughter Elisa. Elisa faced eating issues much of her life, and finally and in despair, she committed suicide at the age of 20. After her death, her parents became aware of a diary she had been keeping, telling of the problems she had been dealing with in respect to her bulimia and depression. She indicated in her diary that she hoped her own story might be helpful in some way to others who were also dealing with eating disorders. The goal of the Elisa Project is to improve awareness of eating disorder issues, provide information about those issues, support individuals who are dealing with eating disorders in their own lives, and work for the development and improvement of programs designed for the prevention and treatment of eating disorders.

One major activity of the project is its prevention curriculum, consisting of classroom presentations on topics such as "The Big Picture" (a general overview of eating disorders), "My Normal Is Not Your Normal: Image Reimagined" (a discussion of body image and self-esteem issues), "Nutrition Up" (information about nutritional issues for healthful living), and

"ED 101" (lectures on the signs, causes, prevention, and treatment of eating disorders). Another important project is the LEAD program, whose name stands for its four elements: learn, empower, accept, and discover. The program is a student-run project that extends over a seven-month period during which participants discuss basic aspects of eating disorders, such as self-esteem, body image, stress, and respect.

The project has also developed a variety of programs to help health-care providers gain a better understanding of the nature, causes, prevention, and treatment of eating disorders. One element of this feature is a group of lectures for professionals on basic information about eating disorders. Another is a Wellness Summit held annually that includes lectures and discussions on eating disorder issues. Toolkits are also available from the project for professionals on eating disorders. The organization also sponsors a group of annual fund-raising events, such as the "life lessons" luncheon, NEDA walks in support of Elisa programs, "Poker with a Purpose" tournament, Esteem Fashion Show (celebrating a positive body image and self-esteem), and the TEP Open Tennis Tournament.

A useful service provided by the Elisa Project is its case management program, whose purpose it is to help clients "navigate your way to health and wellness." This service helps a person to develop advocacy skills with which he or she can help a person "find your own voice" about the problems one faces. It also includes an educational component through which a person can obtain up-to-date, accurate information about eating disorders. The Support and Guidance for Caregivers feature aids friends, family, and loved ones with the knowledge and skills they need to help a person through the difficult process of recovery. The case management also provides assistance with treatment facilities and specific issues about treatment for individuals.

Yet another service provided by the project is its ED Educator Ambassador program. The program offers schools the opportunity to connect with some individual trained in and knowledgeable about eating disorder issues so that students in any particular school will have the opportunity to get on-site assistance.

Galen (129/130? CE–210/216? CE)

From the second to about the seventeenth century, Galen was the preeminent physician in Western culture. In fact, the dominant theory of medicine during that time was often referred to as *Galenic medicine*. Unlike modern medicine, Galenic medicine was seldom based on experimental studies of the human body. Instead, it grew out of careful observations by skilled physicians, who then developed theories as to the causes of health and disease. Galenic medicine was based on the presumption that a balance among four substances (humors) in the human body was responsible for maintaining health. An excess or deficiency of any one humor was the cause of one or another kind of disease. The four humors described in Galenic medicine were black bile, yellow bile, blood, and phlegm.

During his lifetime, Galen wrote about almost every aspect of human health and disease. (Although some works ascribed to Galen may well have been written by other individuals, those individuals may have adopted Galen's name to add credence to their own thoughts and practices. Or later historians may simply have misattributed a work to Galen.) In such a case, it would be remarkable if he did not have something to say about various types of eating disorders, along with his comments about other topics. In the case of obesity, for example, Galen believed that overweight was caused by an excess of blood in the body, a problem that could be cured by bleeding. Galen also took note of disorders in which people ate excessive amounts of food and then voluntarily vomited sometimes to resume eating again. He called the disorder *boulimos*, a term that had actually been in use for centuries to describe the fainting that occurred, usually as the result of exposure to severely cold weather. Since fainting also occurred with binge eating, Galen adopted the older term to describe a condition that is almost always associated with bulimia today. A third eating disorder recognized by Galen was greensickness, in which a person's skin (almost always a woman's) took on a greenish pall, accompanying a morbid dislike of certain types of food, especially meats. The condition today might be thought of as a form of pica because of its emphasis on the ingestion (or rejection) of certain types of food.

Aelius Galenus (also known as Claudius Galenus) was born in Pergamon (or Pergamum), on the western coast of modern-day Turkey, in September of 129 CE. He is most commonly known today simply as Galen, or Galen of Pergamon. Galen's father, Aelius Nicon, was a prosperous architect with a wide-ranging interest in fields such as agriculture, astronomy, literature, mathematics, and philosophy. He hoped that his son would follow a similar career, and the family's financial security certainly allowed this path for the young Galen. As one of the most prominent cities in Greece at the time, Pergamon afforded Galen abundant opportunities for the personalized study of the principal fields of academic pursuit, such as literature, mathematics, and philosophy.

The story is told that the planned trajectory of Galen's life was interrupted when he was about 15 years of age. His father is said to have had a dream in which Asclepius, the Greek god of medicine, appeared to him and foretold that the correct future for his son was a career in medicine. Acting on that dream, Nicon arranged for his son to begin studying with the finest medical teachers then available in Pergamon, which itself was the center of medical teaching in Greece. When Nicon died in 148, Galen inherited his vast fortune, which he used to travel throughout the developed world, studying the various philosophical and medical theories of the day. His travels took him to most of the major Greek centers of learning, including Cilicia, Corinth, Crete, Cyprus, Smyrna, and, most important, the great medical school of Alexandria.

At the conclusion of his journeys in 157, Galen was appointed physician to the gladiators serving the high priest of

Asia in Pergamon. During his four-year stint in this position, he was exposed to and required to treat a host of wounds and illnesses experienced by the gladiators, vastly improving his understanding of the anatomy and physiology of the human body. At the same time, he continued his own studies in medicine and philosophy and worked as a consulting physician to the many visitors coming to Pergamon for treatment.

Galen's tenure in Pergamon ended in 162 when a civil conflict broke out in the region. He decided to move to Rome, where he began to teach his own theory and practice of medicine. His approach to health and disease was considered radical by local physicians, constant disputes occurred, and fearing for the safety of his life, Galen returned to Pergamon. After a few quiet years in his hometown, Galen was recalled to Rome by the emperors Marcus Aurelius and Lucius Verus to serve as physician to the Roman army. He remained in that post until 169, when he was assigned to serve as personal physician to Marcus Aurelius and his son Commodus. The last decade of Galen's life is not well documented, and recent research suggests that his death date may actually be as late as 216, rather than the date of 210 traditionally assigned to that event.

William W. Gull (1816–1890)

In 1873, Gull read two papers before the Clinical Society of London. One of these papers dealt with a condition that he called *anorexia hysterica*, which occurred in (primarily) young women. The condition resulted in their somewhat dramatic wasting away and appearing much older than their biological age. The second paper concerned another condition, which he called the *cretinoid state* that he also observed in certain female patients. In a somewhat remarkable twist of history, the latter paper was received well and became widely regarded among his listeners, while the former paper was largely considered to be irrelevant and was largely ignored, not only by his audience in London but also by scholars of eating disorders to nearly a century thereafter. Indeed, biographies of Gull written after his death and into the twentieth century continued to ignore his treatment of anorexia in favor of the paper on the condition he referred to as *myxoedema*, or "a cretinoid state in adults." Today, Gull's research has earned him the recognition (along with French physician Ernest-Charles Lasègue) as the first person to definitely describe and name the condition now known as anorexia nervosa.

William Withy Gull was born on December 31, 1816, in the town of Colchester, in southeastern England. His father was John Gull, a barge owner and wharfinger (overseer of a wharf), and his mother was Elizabeth (Chilver) Gull. The Gulls had eight children in all, two of whom died in infancy. William was the youngest of the children. Biographies of Gull report that his father was "an honest, upright man, devoted to his children," but his mother was a "remarkable woman," to whom her husband looked for advice in every important matter (Acland 1851). In 1820, the Gull family moved to Thorpe-le-Soken, in Essex, where young William was raised. Seven years later, John Gull died of cholera in London, leaving his children in the sole care of their mother.

In his youth, Gull attended schools in his home parish, one run by two women and the other by a local clergyman. His mother was insistent on his concentrating on his education and required him to spend a certain amount of time on his studies each day. At the age of 15, Gull became a boarder at the clergyman's school, but he stayed only two years. At that point, he later said, he had learned all that the man was able to teach him. After leaving the school, Gull became attached to another school operated by a Mr. Abbott, with whose family he lived during his tenure at the school. During his years with Abbott, Gull was both a student, beginning his studies in more advanced topics, and a teacher of younger students at the school.

At about this time, Gull was imagining that he would like to become a seaman. Those plans were disrupted, however, when he was invited to continue his studies at the local Guy's Hospital. In 1837, the treasurer of the hospital, Benjamin Harrison, took notice of Gull's work and arranged for him to move to London, where he continued his studies at the University of London Medical School. While still studying for his MD degree, Gull also taught a variety of subjects, including anatomy, natural science, and physiology at the hospital. He was granted his bachelor of medicine degree in 1841 and his MD from London in 1846. He then remained at the hospital, continuing his teaching in the biological sciences. At his graduation, Gull was awarded a gold medal for his scholarly accomplishments, the highest honor then available at the university.

After graduating from London, Gull returned to Guy's, where he served as lecturer in physiology and comparative anatomy for the next 10 years. He was then offered the prestigious appointment as Fullerian Professor of Physiology at the Royal Institution, a post he held for two years. In 1848, he was appointed a fellow of the Royal College of Physicians and, at the same time, the post of resident physician at Guy's. Gull held the latter post until 1865, when he resigned because of the demands associated with his private practice.

In 1871, Gull achieved some measure of public adulation when he treated the Prince of Wales, who was then suffering from typhoid fever. In recognition of his work, he was named a baronet a year later by Queen Victoria. At the same time, he was appointed to be a physician to the queen, a post he held until 1887. He then suffered the first of a series of strokes that forced him to greatly reduce his professional work. Although he continued to maintain a reduced practice, he never fully recovered and finally died in London after another stroke on January 29, 1890.

In addition to his appointment as a baronet, Gull received a number of other honors during his life, including honorary degrees by the universities of Cambridge, Edinburgh, and Oxford. He was also selected to deliver the Gulstonian

Lectures before the College of Physicians in 1849, the Hunterian Oration before the Hunterian Society in 1861, the Address on Medicine before the British Medical Association in 1868, and the Harveian Oration before the College of Physicians in 1870.

Charles Ernest Lasègue (1816–1883)

In one of the not-so-rare events in the history of science, Lasègue published a paper in 1873 ("De l'anorexie hystérique" ["Hysterical Anorexia"]) in the *Archives Générales de Médecine* (1: 385–403) on anorexia nervosa in the same year as one by the English physician William Gull (see earlier). The coincidence of the two papers suggests that both men should receive some recognition as the first to describe the condition. (Gull is sometimes given priority because he gave a lecture on the topic, without issuing a formal paper, five years earlier.) Both papers essentially disappeared from the consciousness of researchers for nearly a century, until the study of anorexia once more became a topic of considerable research in the field of mental disorders.

Charles Ernest Lasègue (also given as Ernest Charles Lasègue) was born in Paris on September 5, 1816, to Jacques Antoine Lasègue and Rosalie Charlotte Scholastique Schéricy. His father was employed as both a botanist and librarian by the wealthy French banker and naturalist Jules Paul Benjamin Delessert. Lasègue pursued a traditional course of classical studies at the Lycee Louis-le-Grand, from which he graduated with a degree in letters in 1838. He then stayed on at the school and became a teacher at a modest salary. The salary was so meager, in fact, that he briefly considered opening a bed-and-breakfast in Paris with his mother.

Those plans changed, however, largely because of his blossoming friendship with physiologist Claude Bernard and psychiatrist Bénédict Morel. In fact, Lasègue became involved with some of Bernard's research, assisting him in the treatment of patients with a variety of medical conditions. These experiences led Lasègue to decide that he should continue his studies, now in the field of medicine with a special interest in psychiatry. As a consequence, he enrolled in the Faculté de Médecine at the University of Paris in 1839 and obtained his doctorate there in 1847. On completion of his studies, he was asked by the French government to visit Russia in order to study the epidemic of cholera that was then sweeping the country. During this visit, Lasègue took the opportunity to visit asylums for the mentally disturbed to observe their practices and procedures.

On his return to France, Lasègue was appointed head of a medical clinic at Trousseau, a post he held for two years. During this tenure, he studied for and received his agrégation, the highest level available in the French civil service system. Also in 1853, Lasègue was appointed editor of the medical section of the *Archives générales de médecine*, a post he held until his death 30 years later. Over the next decade, he worked and taught at the Lourcine, La Salpêtrière, Saint Antoine, and Necker hospitals. In 1862, Lasègue was appointed physician-in-chief of the Insane Infirmary at the Paris Prefecture of Police. There he had the opportunity to study a range of men and women accused and/or convicted of criminal activities. He wrote a number of papers on the apparent psychiatric characteristics of the individuals he saw in that position.

In 1869, Lasègue was appointed professor of medicine and general therapeutics at the Hospital de la Pitie, where he remained until his death. He died in Paris on March 20, 1883. Today Lasègue is probably best known as the founder of the concept of folie à deux, in which a delusional disorder is shared by two or more individuals, often members of the same family. The condition is also known today as Lasègue-Falret syndrome. His name is also memorialized in the *Lasègue sign*, a test conducted to determine whether or not a patient has a herniated disc in his or her spine.

National Association for Males with Eating Disorders

The National Association for Males with Eating Disorders was founded in 2006 by Christopher Clark, a man who had eating disorder issues as a high school student and has since recovered. The organization is currently sponsored and supported in part by about a half dozen for-profit companies with programs for the treatment of eating disorders, including the Reasons Eating Disorder Center, Rosewood Centers for Eating Disorders, Rogers Behavioral Health, Fairwinds Treatment Center, and Veritas Collaborative. On its website, the organization provides information about anorexia nervosa, bulimia nervosa, binge eating disorder, and muscle dysphoria, along with a page on myths about male eating disorders. The website also has a good "Get Information" section that provides links to articles and books with special emphasis on eating disorders among males, along with videos devoted to the topic and a list and description of research projects on various aspects of male eating disorders.

National Association of Anorexia Nervosa and Associated Disorders

The National Association of Anorexia Nervosa and Associated Disorders (ANAD) was founded in 1976 by Vivian Hanson Meeham, a nurse at a hospital in Highland Park, Illinois. A few years earlier, Meeham's daughter had been diagnosed with anorexia nervosa, and she decided to search for more information about the disorder. She soon found that no group existed to provide information and support for men and women with the disorders or for their loved ones or concerned friends. She decided to put an advertisement in a local paper that was picked up by a national magazine and was inundated with calls from other individuals across the nation who were also interested in learning more about anorexia. After formalizing these contacts, Meeham founded ANAD as a 501c3 nonprofit organization.

Today, ANAD consists of a number of support groups with special interest and expertise in the areas of therapists, physicians, dentists, psychiatrists, yoga professionals, dietitians and nutritionists, expressive arts therapists, and treatment centers. Information about and location of such groups can be found on the organization's interactive website at http://www.anad .org/our-services/treatment-directory/. The organization also provides a helpline that is available from 9:00 A.M. to 5:00 P.M. on weekdays (Central Time) at (630) 577–1330. The "Find Your Voice with ANAD" online blog also provides individuals with an opportunity to share their issues, problems, and tales of success with others dealing with anorexia. ANAD's annual convention features lectures and discussion groups, along with a variety of exhibits, which deal with all aspects of anorexia nervosa and certain other eating disorders. ANAD also publishes a monthly online newsletter available to anyone interested in the organization's work.

One of the interesting services provided by the organization is the availability of recovery mentors and grocery buddies. A recovery mentor is an individual who has had an eating disorder and recovered from the experience. He or she is available to assist someone struggling with an eating disorder by sharing information and feelings about the experience. ANAD matches recovery mentors with individuals who request such an assistance on the organization's website. A grocery buddy is also someone with experience in eating disorder issues who is matched with someone dealing with an eating disorder condition. He or she accompanies the person shopping to aid him or her in selecting the kinds of foods that will be most helpful in moving on from anorexia, bulimia, or some other eating disorder.

ANAD provides a number of other online services relating to eating disorders, such as an information page on the types and symptoms of eating disorders, statistics on such disorders, and suggestions for helping a friend or loved one with an eating disorder. The Education & Awareness web page has suggestions for school presentations, an educational video, access to the YouTube Recovery Channel, and information on educational partnerships dealing with eating disorders. The website also provides access to some useful educational and training tools that are directed at specific groups, such as mental health-care providers, medical health-care providers, school educators, recovery mentors, grocery buddies, helpline volunteers, and support group leaders.

National Association to Advance Fat Acceptance

The history of the National Association to Advance Fat Acceptance (NAAFA) dates to the mid-1960s when William J. Fabrey had reached the end of his patience with individuals who were rude or condescending to his wife, Joyce, a "very plus-sized woman." In a keynote address to the NAAFA "Big as Texas" in 2001, Fabrey related a number of unhappy experiences to which he and his wife were exposed during their courtship and years of marriage. (Fabrey's speech is available at http://big astexas.tripod.com/2001event/keynote2001.html.) He finally decided that it would be helpful to form a support group of others who, like he and Joyce, were constantly confronted with antiobesity attitudes and comments. He wrote out a constitution for such a group and, with a handful of other supporters, signed the document on June 13, 1969. The organization's current mission statement expresses the goal of "[eliminating] discrimination based on body size and [providing] fat people with the tools for self-empowerment though public education, advocacy, and support."

The core philosophy of NAAFA is that obesity is generally not a personal choice but the result of genetic and other biological factors, as well as environmental influences. This philosophy stands in stark contrast to current social and cultural attitudes that appear to emphasize that "thinness is good," and overweight is a willful neglect of societal standards.

The organization believes that overweight is "one of the last publicly accepted discriminatory practices" ("About Us" 2018) and that fat people have civil rights the same as do other Americans. One objective of the organization is to work to make sure that those rights are acknowledged and respected. Another principal NAAFA belief is that a powerful factor in discrimination against fat people is the $49 billion diet industry, which appears to have a vested interest in maintaining current social attitudes and practices with regard to overweight and obesity.

The NAAFA website is a good source of information about many aspects of overweight and obesity issues. Its "Issues" section, for example, describes manifestations of fat discrimination in education, the workplace, and health-care industry. In addition, the "Education" section of the website offers programs and activities in which one can participate to support the organization's goals and objectives. It reviews the Health at Every Size (HAES) curriculum, developed by NAAFA in collaboration with the Association for Size Diversity and Health (ASDH), as one excellent source for educating students of all ages, from elementary to college, as well as health professionals, about weight perceptions and issues. (An overview of the curriculum is available at https://haescurriculum.com/.)

The "Education" section also has an excellent summary of current and proposed laws dealing with weight issues. Only one state (Michigan) has so far adopted such a law, although similar legislation has also been enacted in a number of cities, including Binghamton, New York; Madison, Wisconsin; San Francisco; Santa Cruz, California; Urbana, Illinois; and Washington, D.C. Information on international legal events relating to weight issues can also be found at this site. Another NAAFA program is focused on the increasingly serious problem of weight bullying, in which children whose weight does not correspond to societal expectations are subjected to bullying by their peers. The organization has developed fact sheets on bullying and on ways to end the practice, as well as an exhaustive and detailed toolkit for use with children of all ages (available at https://www.naafaonline

.com/dev2/about/Brochures/NAAFA_Child_Advocacy_Tool kit.pdf). The "Education" website also has links to print and online articles, books, and organizations, with further information on weight issues, as well as links to resources on topics such as size acceptance, size positive, fat art and gifts, men's clothing, nonclothing, online community, travel, women's clothing, and health and wellness.

National Eating Disorder Association

The National Eating Disorder Association (NEDA) was founded in 2001 as a result of the merger of what were then the two oldest and largest eating disorder organizations, Eating Disorders Awareness & Prevention and the American Anorexia Bulimia Association. The goal of the organization is to provide assistance to individuals and families having to deal with any type of eating disorder while at the same time working to improve prevention, cures, and quality care. The organization is run by a board of directors with 19 members and advised by a group of 7 senior advisers. The organization's home office is in New York City and can be reached by e-mail at info@National EatingDisorders.org or by telephone at (212) 575-6200. NEDA also offers a toll-free hotline for confidential assistance at (800) 931-2237.

NEDA carries on a very ambitious program of services for people interested in or dealing with eating disorder issues. Elements of its program include the following:

- An online eating disorder screening tool, in which individuals can provide basic information about their current status and receive feedback as to their status with regard to eating disorders. The tool provides an automated answer that can recommend further steps in a treatment option.
- The toll-free helpline, which is available Monday through Thursday from 9:00 A.M. to 9:00 P.M. and Friday from 9:00 A.M. to 5:00 P.M. (EST) (not available on holidays).

- Contact information for existing eating disorder groups and individuals and organizations currently conducting on some aspect of eating disorders.

- Access to so-called navigators, with special expertise in dealing with eating disorders, who work with individuals dealing with eating disorder issues. They may help a person to find resources, treatment options, and support groups; answer basic questions about eating disorders; offer hope and encouragement; assist with insurance questions and issues; and provide a list of organizations that can assist with a person's individual problems.

- Provide access to networks of parents, children, siblings, partners, and friends of individuals dealing with eating disorders. A discrete part of the organization's web page provides specialized information about each of these specific groups.

- Maintain a loss support network designed for individuals who have lost a loved one to an eating disorder. An opportunity is provided to volunteer to serve on the network or to seek comfort and advice from someone who has had experience with such an issue.

- Support an annual National Eating Disorders Awareness Week and NEDA Walks designed to educate the general public about eating disorder issues and raise funds for the organization's operations.

- Provide a Legislative Advocacy portal through which interested individuals can become active in working for the education of legislators about eating disorders and gaining additional funding for research, education, and other aspects of the NEDA agenda.

- Sponsor the Feeding Hope Fund for Clinical Research, which solicits funds to be used exclusively for the support of research projects on eating disorders.

- Participates in the Body Project, a dissonance-based project in which participants explore body images in the current mass media, with the goal of retreating from an unrealistic "thin-body" image that may be at the base of their own eating disorder.

- Coordinates the NEDA Network, which consists of a number of independent like-minded organizations. Among the members of the organization are the American Anorexia and Bulimia Association, Eating Disorder Foundation, the Elisa Project, Ophelia's Place, Project Heal, and Realize Your Beauty.

Probably the most valuable service of the organization for the general public is the "General Information" and "By Eating Disorder" sections of its website. These sections provide very useful information on eating disorders, in general, such as risk factors, warning signs, health consequences, diagnosis, and treatment (General Information), as well as detailed information on all of the currently recognized eating disorders. The website also provides an excellent and extensive glossary of terms related to eating disorders and toolkits designed specifically for parents, educators, and coaches and athletic trainers. Each toolkit provides relevant detailed information about topics such as characteristics and causes of eating disorders, suggestions for assisting and supporting individuals with a disorder, methods of treatment, and information about insurance for treatment programs.

National Eating Disorder Information Centre

The National Eating Disorder Information Centre (NEDIC) was founded in 1985, following an earlier study by the Health League of Canada of national needs in the area of eating disorders. The mission of NEDIC was to focus on eating disorders and how the choices that women make are affected by overall social and cultural norms and practices. The organization was funded for two years by the Health League, after which support was provided on a temporary basis by the Toronto General

Hospital with funding from the Ontario Ministry of Health. In 1993, that funding became permanent, and NEDIC is now a constituent part of the Toronto Hospital Eating Disorders Program. The center espouses a strong feminist philosophy that is based in a belief that a person's eating habits are strongly influenced by social and cultural factors and not by a person's biological makeup. It does not refer individuals to treatment centers with specialized diets to aid them in overcoming eating disorders but works, instead, to help them build a self-affirming and strong personal outlook on their life. An additional goal of the program is to help change social attitudes about a person's body shape and size, overcoming unfair and harmful views as to what constitutes a body that is "too fat," "too thin," or "abnormal" in any other way.

NEDIC's work is organized into three major areas: outreach and education, direct client support, and additional programs. The goal of the outreach and education arm of the program is to promote critical thinking skills and a healthy lifestyle as a way of becoming better informed about the nature of eating disorders and the steps that can be taken to prevent such disorders. This goal is accomplished through the dissemination of information about eating disorders, self-esteem, body image, and related issues. The organization works toward this goal through presentations, workshops, panel discussions, and webinars designed for schools, community groups, and professionals in health care and education. NEDIC is also involved in education through its national Eating Disorders Awareness Week, held annually, and the International No Diet Day.

The NEDIC direct client support program consists of two elements: a toll-free helpline, claimed to be the only dedicated telephone resource providing support for individuals with eating disorders and information about resources to which such individuals can turn for additional assistance, and a national directory of more than 600 providers who offer assistance with eating disorders.

One of the additional programs of the organization is a curriculum program for grades 4 through 8 on self-esteem and body image issues that may contribute to the development of eating disorders. The program is available at no charge at http://beyondimages.ca/. A second additional program is called the Be You Challenge for Girl Guide groups throughout the nation. (Girl Guides are similar to Girl Scouts in the United States.) Discrete Be You Challenge programs are available at each level of the Girl Guides program. NEDIC also sponsors a biennial conference for professionals in the field of eating disorders on self-esteem, body image, and related topics.

An especially useful service available on the NEDIC website is its "Know the Facts" section, which provides detailed information on a range of topics, including "Food and Weight Preoccupation"; "Body Image and Self-Esteem"; "Social, Cultural, and Biological Influences"; "Treatment, Support, and Recovery"; "Prevention and Health Promotion"; "Definitions"; "Statistics, Pro-Eating Disorder Websites"; "Information Resources"; and "Frequently Asked Questions." Another section, known as "Give and Get Help," is another source of help. It includes discrete pages on Help for You, Help for Friends and Family, Understanding Treatment Options, Service Provider Directory, Prevention and Health Promotion, Personal Stories, and NEDIC Webinar Recordings.

National Eating Disorders Collaboration

The National Eating Disorders Collaboration (NEDC) is an initiative established in 2009 and funded by the Australian government that brings together experts in mental health, public health, public health promotion, education, research, the media, and others concerned with issues of eating disorders for the purpose of developing a nationally consistent program for the prevention and treatment of eating disorders. Its primary objectives are to

- provide or facilitate access to helpful, evidence-based information to young people and their families on the prevention and management of eating disorders and healthy eating;
- promote a consistent, evidence-based national approach to eating disorders;
- develop and assist in implementing a comprehensive national strategy to communicate appropriate evidence-based messages to schools, the media, and health-service providers.

As explained on the NEDC website, the methods by which the organization expects to achieve these objectives are as follows:

1. Works collaboratively to develop eating disorders knowledge

   - Builds, engages and supports a collaboration of experts, key stakeholders and people with an interest in eating disorders
   - Builds intersectoral and interdisciplinary coordination and evidence sharing on eating disorders and fosters professional learning

2. Promotes evidence-based information

   - Provides or facilitates access to helpful evidence-based information to young people and their families on the prevention and management of eating disorders and healthy eating
   - Provides access to evidence-based information on the prevention and management of eating disorders, including identifying the best information available to help health practitioners and other professionals in the treatment, management and prevention of eating disorders

3. Develops and promotes consistent national standards

- Promotes a consistent evidence-based national approach to eating disorders
- Analyses existing resources and approaches, including their evidence base
- Builds/enhances and assists in raising awareness of a national evidence-based framework for the prevention and management of eating disorders
- Identifies gaps in the services and information available to people with eating disorders and their families

4. Communicates the evidence

- Develops and assists in implementing a comprehensive national strategy to communicate appropriate evidence-based messages to schools, the media and health service providers
- Identifies and works with key stakeholders and established initiatives to raise awareness of evidence-based approaches for the early intervention of eating disorders. (From http://www.nedc.com.au/about-the-nedc)

The NEDC website is one of the most useful online resources available to individuals interested in learning more about eating disorders and/or who are looking for aid in dealing with their own eating disorder issues. One section, "Eating Disorders Explained," provides basic information on all of the fundamental issues related to eating disorders, including detailed explanations of the major disorders, risk factors for eating disorders, the question of body image as a factor in the development of eating disorders, prevention and treatment, special issues for males, the problem of eating disorders in Australia, and myths about eating disorders. Another valuable web page is called the Knowledge Hub. It includes reports on the latest research on eating disorders, a resource directory, a list of NEDC publications, and a free monthly e-bulletin newsletter summarizing recent research, information for professionals in the field, and upcoming events.

The "Treatment and Recovery" section of the website provides detailed information about all aspects of treatment, such as a description as to what takes place during treatment programs, methods that are used, likely costs and payment for services, complementary options for treatment, stages of change, and the possibility of relapse and recurrence of a disorder.

In order to achieve its objectives, NEDC has also developed a wide variety of learning and counseling resources that are available for downloading at no cost. Currently available fact sheets deal with other specified feeding and eating disorders, bulimia nervosa, binge eating disorder, anorexia nervosa, disordered eating and dieting, body image, and eating disorders in males. Infographics on Eating Disorders in Australia, Myths Busted, Seven Tips for Families and Carers, Guys Get Eating Disorders Too, Seven Tips for Improving Body Image, and Getting Help for Someone You're Worried About are also available. A number of resources are aimed at specific groups interested in eating disorders, such as health professionals (e.g., "Pharmacy and Eating Disorders" and "Dentistry and Eating Disorders"), teachers and schools ("Eating Disorders in Schools: Prevention, Early Identification, and Response"), sport and fitness professionals ("Eating Disorders in Sport and Fitness: Prevention, Early Identification, and Response"), and families and caregivers (e.g., "Caring for Someone with an Eating Disorder").

Obesity Action Coalition

Until relatively recently, no specific organization existed to represent the millions of Americans who deal with the issue of obesity. Then, in 2005, at a congressional hearing on the subject, one legislator raised the question as to who it was that did represent obese Americans. When no answer was forthcoming, activists interested in obesity designed to form such an organization. And thus arose today's Obesity Action Coalition (OAC), whose mission it is to "[give] a voice to the individual affected by the disease of obesity and [help] individuals along their journey toward better health through education, advocacy and support." Today, OAC claims a membership of more than 54,000 individuals who are committed to this goal. Memberships in the organization are available for $20 for individuals and $500 or $1,000 for institutional memberships, depending on the level of commitment. Membership benefits include subscriptions to the organization's two regular publications, its quarterly magazine, *Your Weight Matters*, and its monthly newsletter, "OAC Members Make a Difference." The organization's monthly online newsletter, "Obesity Action Alert," is available at no charge to any interested party, member or not.

A core component of OAC is a group of committees that carry out the organization's administration and programmatic chores. The former includes the executive, nominating, convention, membership, revenue generating, and long-range planning committees. The latter group includes the education, access to care, and visibility committee, along with the weight bias task force. The four committees coordinate their activities with the goal of providing a better understanding of the nature of obesity and issues that may surround the condition for both the general public and those dealing with obesity itself. Each committee also has its own special emphasis. The weight bias task force, for example, concentrates on identifying examples of weight bias in the general media and working through OAC to combat those biases.

An important function of the organization's website is education about obesity issues for both members and the general public. It includes helpful sections on the meaning of "obesity" and "severe obesity," ways of measuring weight, medical and other conditions related to obesity, the problems of childhood obesity, measuring weight in children, and the stigma faced by obese children. National and regional meetings are also an important part of the organization's educational and support program. In addition to the annual convention, it sponsors local and regional Your Weight Matters conferences on obesity issues. OAC has also developed and distributes a large variety of print materials (also available online at no charge; some also available in Spanish) on topics such as "Understanding Obesity"; "Understanding Severe Obesity"; "Understanding Childhood Obesity"; "Understanding Obesity Stigma"; "Excess Weight and Health Guidebook and Video"; "Excess Weight and Your Health—A Guide to Effective, Healthy Weight Loss"; "Weight-Loss Options"; "Obesity and Type 2 Diabetes"; "Understanding Excess Weight and Its Role in Type 2 Diabetes"; "Understanding Prediabetes and Excess Weight"; "Obesity-Related Diseases"; "Obesity and Cancer"; "Obesity and Eating Disorders"; "Obesity and Heart Disease"; "Obesity and Hypertension"; "Obesity and Lipid Issues"; "Obesity and Osteoarthritis"; "Obesity and Stroke"; "OAC Insurance Guide"; "Working with Your Insurance Provider: A Guide to Seeking Weight-Loss Surgery"; "Weight Gain and Your Joints"; "Weight Gain and Joint Pain"; and "Can My Weight Make My Joint Pain Worse?"

A critical aspect of the OAC program is its advocacy initiative, which consists of many elements. Its "Getting Started" website, for example, provides a number of suggestions for ways in which individuals can become engaged in the effort to educate legislators and the general public about issues surrounding obesity. The "Public Policy" section brings together all of the letters and other statements formally made by the organization to legislators and others in decision-making positions. The "Health Policy Agenda" is a document that summarizes the OAC's position on a number of obesity-related issues, such as obesity discrimination, treatment of obesity, insurances policies, obesity issues in the workplace, governmental bodies an obesity, obesity in schools, and marketing and obesity.

The website "Legislative Action Center" brings together summaries of pending state and federal legislation related to obesity, with links to individuals who can be contacted and lobbied on each topic. The organization's State Advocacy Resource program focuses more specifically on problems at the state legislative and regulatory levels. In support of this objective, the OAC website has an exhaustive range of resources that can be used at the state level, including fact sheets for each state, state guides, and resources for working at the state level.

Overeaters Anonymous

Overeaters Anonymous (OA) was founded by Roxanne S. in 1960. (As with Alcohols Anonymous, Drug Addicts Anonymous, Sex Addicts Anonymous, and similar groups, first names are used only in describing individual members.) Two years earlier, Roxanne had attended a Gamblers Anonymous (GA) meeting with a friend and realized that the program offered by GA was one that might help with her own overeating issues. At the time, she weighed 152 pounds and stood 5 feet 2 inches tall. As she continued to gain weight, she came across a neighbor who was dealing with similar problems and, before long, the two of them had found yet a third woman also dealing with issues of overeating. The three women announced the initial meeting of OA in Los Angeles on January 19, 1960. That organization has grown to consist of about 6,500 individual groups in 75 countries with over 60,000 members. OA claims to have a concern for all types of eating disorders, including anorexia, bulimia, and binge eating, as well as overeating itself.

Overeaters Anonymous subscribes to a 12-step program similar to the one originated by AA. The 12 steps recognized by OA members such changes as admitting that one is powerless over the problem of overeating, accepting the fact that a power greater than oneself is needed to solve the problem, making a moral inventory of oneself, turning one's life over to God or some other higher power, making amends for harm that has occurred to others because of overeating issues, and recognizing new insights as a result of this process. The 12-step program relies heavily on a willingness to hand one's problem over to God or a higher power. But OA points out that this emphasis need to deter individuals who are atheists or agnostics. The organization says that OA members have a wide range of spiritual beliefs that allow them to adapt the group's principle to their own plan of action for dealing with overeating and other eating disorders.

The tools available to OA members are similar to those of other 12-step groups. They include a plan for dealing with one's problem (e.g., overeating), finding and working with a sponsor, attending meetings regularly, putting one's thought down on paper, reading more about the issue of overeating, and developing a personal action plan to direct one's steps in overcoming the overeating issue.

One of the critical functions of OA is to help people dealing with eating disorders to find and join local groups of the organization. Another basic service provided by the organization is access to a wide variety of educational and support materials, such as a quarterly print and online newsletter, "A Step Ahead," and podcasts of virtual workshops dealing with procedural topics (e.g., the importance of abiding by the 12-step process), as well as the sharing of experience among members of the group; looking for and serving as a sponsor; ways of contributing to OA; the importance of anonymity; the importance of each of the 12 steps that form the basis of OA; members in relapse; eating plans; tools of recovery; and interviews with members who have especially valuable stories to tell. The organization's *Lifeline* magazine is available to members and is touted as an "indispensable meeting-on-the-go" that one can carry at all times for information and encouragement.

Project HEAL

The idea for Project HEAL originated in 2006 when two young women, Liana Rosenman and Kristina Saffran, both

13 years old at the time, met during treatment for their eating disorders. They supported each other through the treatment process and eventually decided to form an organization to help individuals deal specifically with the problem of funding for eating disorder treatments. Their decision reflected the reality that eating disorder treatments can be very expensive, costing as much as $30,000 per month, an expense that some insurance companies do not cover in their normal policies. As a consequence, many men and women and boys and girls, who would otherwise benefit from a treatment program, are unable to enroll in one.

Another factor in the decision to create the project was the girls' realization that, even after their cure, they were encountering peers who also needed treatment or, in many cases, simply did not know very much about eating disorders. They decided that they "wanted to do something to change the conversation." A final factor in the decision to form an organization was the fact that during their treatments, the girls often felt that they were in a hopeless situation. They came to understand that one element in a successful treatment program is the belief that life will get better after treatment, and it is possible to once more lead a "normal" life. One of the most powerful features of the Project HEAL website is the individual stories written by Liana and Kristina of their own struggles with eating disorders and how their treatment experiences changed their outlook on life.

Project HEAL is administered and operated by various types of boards and individual contributors, including a board of directors, clinical advisory board, advisory board, junior advisory board, "champions," and "ambassadors." The organization has about 40 local chapters in 21 states, the District of Columbia, and Australia and Canada. The primary purpose of the chapters is to raise funds for the project's grant program, with educational outreach a secondary goal.

The goal of Project HEAL is to make grants available to individuals for eating disorder treatments who would not otherwise be able to afford those treatments. Funds for those grants come from individual donations in any amount that are used to fund a specific aspect of treatment (e.g., a one-hour consultation with a nutritionist) or a complete series of treatments. Anyone wishing to participate in the program may apply for a grant on the organization's website at https://www.theprojecttheal.org/memorial-treatment-grants-1/.

Although the project's website is devoted primarily to money-raising and grant-making issues, it also contains some additional useful information. The "Press" page of the site, for example, provides links to a number of presentations on the Internet, in television and motion pictures, and in the print media about eating disorder issues.

Adolphe Quetelet (1796–1874)

Quetelet is probably best known today for his invention of a system for measuring a person's "healthy" body mass, known as the body mass index (BMI). This measure is calculated by dividing a person's body mass by his or her height.

Lambert Adolphe Jacques Quetelet was born in Ghent, France (now Belgium), on February 22, 1796, to Anne-Françoise Vandervelde and François-Augustin-Jacques-Henri Quetelet. His father was an adventurous man who traveled to England to gain British citizenship. While there, he was hired as secretary to a Scottish nobleman, with whom he traveled throughout Europe. He finally settled in Ghent, where he became employed by the city. He died in Ghent in 1803 when his son, Adolphe, was only seven years old.

Quetelet received his formal education at the Lyceé de Gent, where he excelled in mathematics, earning prizes in both algebra and geometry. In addition to his mathematical studies, however, Quetelet became interested in a number of other subjects, an interest that was reflected in the fact, according to his biographer Garabed Eknoyan, that he "published poetry, exhibited his paintings, studied sculpture, co-authored the libretto of an opera and translated Byron and Schiller into French" (Eknoyan 2007). After graduating from the Lyceé, Quetelet spent a year teaching at a private college in Audernarde. He then returned to Ghent to continue his teaching career. In 1817, he left teaching to continue his studies at the newly created University of Ghent, where he studied mathematics under Jean Guillaume Garnier. He was also hired to teach under Garnier, a position that, he argued, should excuse him from the normal series of examinations and go directly to the defense of his thesis. He was given approval for this plan of action and was granted his doctorate in mathematics at Ghent in 1819.

After receiving his doctorate, Quetelet was appointed as a teacher of mathematics at the Brussels Athenaeum. Now intrigued also by the subject of astronomy, Quetelet petitioned the government to consider constructing an observatory in Belgium. To promote that objective, he requested and received permission to travel to Paris to continue his studies in astronomy. There, he worked not only with leading figures in the field, such as François Arago and Alexis Bouvard, but also with prominent mathematicians of the day, including Joseph Fourier, Siméon Poisson, and Pierre Laplace. From these men, Quetelet learned the fundamentals of the new field of statistics and probability, in which he soon became proficient. The topic was of considerable significance to nearly all aspects of mathematics and the physical sciences, but Quetelet envisioned another quite different application in the field of the social sciences. He came to believe that not only could the behavior of particles and events be described by the laws of probability, but so could the properties and behavior of humans.

Quetelet presented his ideas about this topic, which he called *social physics*, in what is probably his most important book, *Sur l'homme et le développement de ses facultés, ou Essai de physique sociale* (*On Man and the Development of His Faculties, or Essays on Social Physics*), published in 1835. In the book, he posits the notion of "the average man," an ideal image of a human with average height, average weight, average head circumference, average arm length, and so on. These averages could be determined, Quetelet pointed out, simply by obtaining the relevant measurements of a large number of individuals and then expressing those measurements as probabilities in the form of a probability curve (the well-known Bell Curve). The closer one fell to the middle of that curve, the more "average" (more "normal") that person was. Individuals who fell at the tails of the curve were less average and, therefore, "less normal." Depending on the characteristic being measured, these outliers could then be diagnosed as physically or mentally abnormal, a procedure of particular interest in determining individuals who might fall outside the normal on moral traits and, thus, were more likely to become criminal. As a way of measuring the body structure of the average person, Quetelet developed the BMI. That measure is still used today to describe body structures and to classify individuals who are not "average," "abnormal," "overweight," or "obese."

After completing his studies in Paris, Quetelet returned to Belgium, where he was appointed professor of higher mathematics at the Athenaeum. He also continued to work toward the development of the observatory he had envisioned. In 1827, he was given permission to start selecting instruments for such an observatory and then spent more than three years visiting similar installations in England, Scotland, Ireland, Holland, Germany, Italy, and Sicily. In 1832, Quetelet was appointed director of the new observatory in Brussels. He held that post only one year before accepting the post of secretary of the Royal Belgian Academy of Sciences, a position he retained until his death 40 years later. A stroke that he suffered in 1855 reduced his ability to maintain an active life in academia, although he continued to serve the academy and carry on some teaching and research projects until just prior to his death in Brussels on February 17, 1874.

During his life, Quetelet received a number of honors, including election to the British Royal Academy, the Royal Institute of the Netherlands, the Royal Society of Edinburgh, and

the Royal Swedish Academy of Sciences. He was also instrumental in creation of the statistical section of the Royal Society, a body that later became the Royal Statistical Society. He
has been memorialized with the name of a lunar crater in his
honor, 1239 Queteleta.

Eric Stice (1967–)

Eric Stice is one of the leading researchers in the field of eating
disorders in the United States. He has written 6 books, 14 book
chapters, and more than 200 scientific articles in refereed journals. He has also received nearly 30 grants for his research on
eating disorder and related topics, such as the etiology of bulimia, the effectiveness of various types of treatment programs,
the evaluation of cognitive dissonance in the treatment of eating disorders, risk factors for bulimia, depression prevention in
high-risk adolescents, illicit drug addiction, neural substrates
of dieting, contributing factors in the development of obesity,
and cognitive dissonance treatments for obesity. In 2012, he
founded, with Carolyn Becker, the Body Project, a program
using cognitive dissonance to aid young women to "resist cultural pressures to conform to the appearance ideal standard of
female beauty and reduce their pursuit of unrealistic bodies"
("The Body Project" 2018).

Eric Stice was born in San Jose, California, on September 6,
1967. He attended the University of Oregon, from which he
received his BS in 1989. He then matriculated at Arizona
State University, which awarded him his MA and PhD in
clinical psychology in 1992 and 1996, respectively. During
his final year at Arizona State University, he also served as
a psychology intern in the Department of Psychiatry at the
University of California at San Diego. He then completed
his postdoctoral studies at the department of psychiatry at
Stanford University.

In 1998, Stice was offered the position of assistant professor of psychology at the University of Texas at Austin. He was

later promoted to associate professor in 2002 and to research professor in 2004 at Texas, a post he held until 2010. In 2003, Stice also accepted an offer to serve as senior scientist at the Oregon Research Institute in Eugene, where he is still employed. Over the past two decades, he has also held a number of other academic appointments, such as visiting assistant professor in psychiatry at Stanford, visiting fellow in psychiatry at Oxford University (England), visiting assistant professor at the University of Washington, courtesy research associate at the University of Oregon, Erskine Fellow in the Department of Psychology at the University of Canterbury in New Zealand, and scientific director in the Department of Medical and Clinical Psychology at the Darnall Army Medical Hospital at Fort Hood, Texas.

Among his honors and awards are election to Phi Beta Kappa and Psi Chi honor societies, Junior Scholar Award from the Mortar Board Honor Society, Dean's List and Dean's Scholar List at the University of Oregon, and Distinguished Scientific Award for Early Career Contributions to Psychopathology of the American Psychological Association. He has served on the editorial boards of the *Journal of Abnormal Psychology*, *Behavior Therapy*, *Psychology of Women Quarterly*, *Journal of Consulting and Clinical Psychology*, *International Journal of Eating Disorders*, *Psychological Bulletin*, and *Psychology of Addictive Behaviors*.

Stice is married to Heather Shaw, a major contributor to the Body Project and to a number of other research projects on eating disorders.

Albert J. Stunkard (1922–2014)

Stunkard was a pioneer in the study of overweight and obesity, as well as other types of eating disorders. He is widely credited with having reframed researchers' and the general public's view of the nature of obesity, showing that the condition has a significant genetic component and is not primarily a matter of poor willpower. Stunkard was also the first researcher to describe a condition known as *night-eating syndrome*, in which a person consumes excessive amounts of food during the evening hours. He later defined a variation of the condition, in which excessive amounts of eating, *binge eating disorder*, occur but not exclusively at night. At his death in 2014, Stunkard was recognized by a number of his colleagues for the significant import of his work, with one colleague telling the *New York Times* that "In the family tree of our work [obesity research], Stunkard would be at the very top" (Vitello 2014).

Albert J. Stunkard (often known as "Mickey") was born in New York City on February 7, 1922. His mother was Frances Klank Stunkard, a librarian, and his father was Horace Stunkard, professor of biology at New York University. Stunkard earned his bachelor's degree from Yale University in 1943 and his MD from Columbia University two years later. On completing his academic work, Stunkard took a position as an army physician in Japan, which was then being occupied by the United States. His experience in Japan inspired a lifelong interest and involvement with both obesity research and Buddhism, a faith he held throughout his life.

In 1948, Stunkard returned to the United States, where he served a three-year residency in psychiatry at Johns Hopkins University. He then moved to the College of Physicians and Surgeons at Columbia (1951–1953) and the Cornell Medical College in Manhattan (1953–1956). In 1957, he accepted an appointment as associate professor at the University of Pennsylvania, an institution with which he remained affiliated for the rest of his academic career. His long tenure at Pennsylvania was interrupted in 1973 for a three-year period of service at the Stanford University Center for the Study of Behavioral Sciences. After his tenure at Stanford, Stunkard returned to Pennsylvania, where he served as professor of psychiatry until his retirement in 1997, after which he received the designation of emeritus professor at Pennsylvania.

Among the honors and awards given to Stunkard were the Menninger Award of the American College of Physicians,

Lifetime Achievement Award of the Academy for Eating Disorders, Rhoda and Bernard Sarnat International Prize in Mental Health of the National Academy of Medicine, and Joseph Goldberger Award in Clinical Nutrition of the American Medical Association. He was twice honored with the Annual Prize Research of the American Psychiatric Association and was awarded with an honorary MD from the University of Edinburgh. In 2007, the University of Pennsylvania created the Albert J. Stunkard Weight Management Program, and in 2015, the Obesity Society created the Friends of Albert (Mickey) Skunard Lifetime Achievement Award in his honor.

References

"About Us." 2018. NAAFA. https://www.naafaonline.com/dev2/about/index.html. Accessed on November 28, 2018.

Acland, Theodore Dyke, ed. 1851. *A Collection of the Published Writings of William Withey Gull, Bart., M.D., F.E.S.* London: The New Sydenham Society. https://ia600207.us.archive.org/1/items/cu31924011938879/cu31924011938879.pdf. Accessed on November 28, 2018.

"The Body Project." 2018. UCLA Student Health Education & Promotion. https://www.healtheducation.ucla.edu/the-body-project. Accessed on November 28, 2018.

Eknoyan, Garabed. 2007. "Adolphe Quetelet (1796–1874)—The Average Man and Indices of Obesity." *Nephrology Dialysis Transplantation.* 23(1): 48.

"Papers of Hilde Bruch." 1985. http://docplayer.net/57191510-Papers-of-hilde-bruch.html. Accessed on November 28, 2018.

Vitello, Paul. 2014. "Dr. Albert J. Stunkard, Destigmatizer of Fat, Dies at 92." *New York Times.* https://www.nytimes.com/2014/07/21/us/21stunkard.html. Accessed on November 28, 2018.

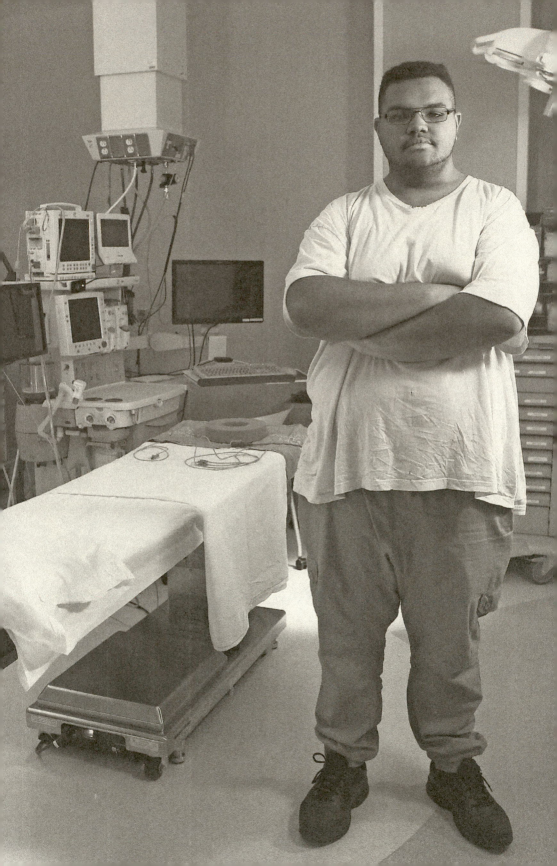

One way to learn about eating disorder issues is through an examination of laws, regulations, court cases, reports, and other documents dealing with the topic. Data and statistics about eating disorders can also provide an insight into the nature of the problem. This chapter provides some basic data about prevalence and incidence of eating disorders in the United States, along with selections from documents that can provide some insights into eating disorders and the issues that surround the topic.

Data

Table 5.1   Prevalence of Overweight, Obese, and Extreme Obesity in the United States, 1988–2014 (percentage of population, aged 20–74)

Period	Total Population			Men			Women		
	Over-weight	Obese	Extremely Obese	Over-weight	Obese	Extremely Obese	Over-weight	Obese	Extremely Obese
1960–1962	31.5	13.4	0.9	38.7	10.7	0.3	24.7	15.8	1.4
1971–1974	32.7	14.5	1.3	41.7	12.1	0.6	24.3	16.6	2.0
1976–1980	32.1	15.0	.1.4	39.9	12.7	0.4	24.9	17.0	2.2
1988–1994	32.6	23.2	3.0	40.3	20.5	1.8	25.1	25.9	4.1
1999–2000	33.6	30.9	5.0	39.2	27.7	3.3	28.0	34.0	6.6
2001–2002	34.4	31.2	5.4	41.5	28.3	3.9	27.3	34.1	6.8

(Continued)

Travion Shinault, a patient at Children's Hospital Colorado in Aurora, hopes that he can still continue his passion for cooking and food after having bariatric surgery. Staff at the hospital were working with Shinault, then only 19, to control his portions and choose healthier food. (RJ Sangosti/ The Denver Post via Getty Images)

Table 5.1   (Continued)

Period	Total Population			Men			Women		
	Over-weight	Obese	Extremely Obese	Over-weight	Obese	Extremely Obese	Over-weight	Obese	Extremely Obese
2003–2004	33.4	32.9	5.1	39.4	31.7	3.0	27.3	34.0	7.3
2005–2006	32.2	35.1	6.2	39.7	33.8	4.3	24.7	36.3	7.9
2007–2008	33.6	34.3	6.0	39.4	32.5	4.4	27.9	36.2	7.6
2009–2010	32.7	36.1	6.6	38.0	35.9	4.6	27.5	36.1	8.5
2011–2012	33.3	35.3	6.6	37.3	33.9	4.5	29.5	36.6	8.6
2013–2014	31.9	38.2	8.1	38.2	35.5	5.7	25.8	41.0	10.5

Source: "Prevalence of Overweight, Obesity, and Extreme Obesity among Adults Aged 20 and Over: United States, 1960–1962 through 2013–2014." 2016. Centers for Disease Control and Prevention, Table 1. https://www.cdc.gov/nchs/data/hestat/obesity_adult_13_14/obesity_adult_13_14.htm. Accessed on April 6, 2017.

Table 5.2   Prevalence of Overweight and Obesity among Children and Adolescents Aged 2–19 Years, by Sex: United States, 1971–1974 through 2013–2014 (percentage of population)

Period	Total Population		Boys		Girls	
	Over-weight	Obese	Over-weight	Obese	Over-weight	Obese
1971–1974	10.2	5.2	10.3	5.3	10.1	5.1
1976–1980	9.2	5.5	9.4	5.4	9.0	5.6
1988–1994	13.0	10.0	12.6	10.2	13.4	9.8
1999–2000	14.2	13.9	15.0	14.0	13.4	13.8
2001–2002	14.6	15.4	14.2	16.4	15.0	14.3
2003–2004	16.5	17.1	16.6	18.2	16.3	16.0
2005–2006	14.6	15.4	14.7	15.9	14.6	14.9
2007–2008	14.8	16.8	14.3	17.7	15.4	15.9
2009–2010	14.9	16.9	14.4	18.6	15.4	15.0
2011–2012	14.9	16.9	15.4	16.7	14.5	17.2
2013–2014	16.2	17.2	16.4	17.2	16.0	17.1

Source: Fryar, Cheryl D., Margaret D. Carroll, and Cynthia L. Ogden. 2016. "Prevalence of Overweight and Obesity among Children and Adolescents Aged 2–19 Years: United States, 1963–1965 through 2013–2014." National Center for Health Statistics, Table 1. https://www.cdc.gov/nchs/data/hestat/obesity_child_13_14/obesity_child_13_14.pdf. Accessed on April 6, 2017.

Table 5.3 Prevalence of Obesity among Children and Adolescents Aged 2–19 Years, by Sex and Age: United States, 1963–1965 through 2013–2014

Period	Total Population			Boys			Girls		
	2–5 Years	6–11 Years	12–19 Years	2–5 Years	6–11 Years	12–19 Years	2–5 Years	6–11 Years	12–19 Years
1971–1974	5.0	4.0	6.1	5.0	4.3	6.1	4.9	3.6	6.2
1976–1980	5.0	6.5	5.0	4.7	6.6	4.8	5.3	6.4	5.3
1988–1994	7.2	11.3	10.5	6.2	11.6	11.3	8.2	11.0	9.7
1999–2000	10.3	15.1	14.8	9.5	15.8	14.8	11.2	14.3	14.8
2001–2002	10.6	16.2	16.7	10.7	17.5	17.6	10.5	14.8	15.7
2003–2004	13.9	18.8	17.4	15.1	19.9	18.2	12.7	17.6	16.4
2005–2006	10.7	15.1	17.8	10.4	16.2	18.2	11.0	14.1	17.3
2007–2008	10.1	19.6	18.1	9.3	21.2	19.3	10.9	18.0	16.8
2009–2010	12.1	18.0	18.4	14.4	20.1	19.6	9.6	15.7	17.1
2011–2012	8.4	17.7	20.5	9.5	16.4	20.3	7.2	19.1	20.7
2013–2014	9.4	17.4	20.6	8.8	18.8	19.8	10.0	15.9	21.4

Source: Fryar, Cheryl D., Margaret D. Carroll, and Cynthia L. Ogden. 2016. "Prevalence of Overweight and Obesity among Children and Adolescents Aged 2–19 Years: United States, 1963–1965 through 2013–2014." National Center for Health Statistics, Table 2. https://www.cdc.gov/nchs/data/hestat/obesity_child_13_14/obesity_child_13_14.pdf. Accessed on April 6, 2017.

Table 5.4 Prevalence of Obesity among Children and Adolescents Aged 2–19 Years, by Sex and Ethnicity: United States, 1963–1965 through 2013–2014

Period	Boys					Girls				
	White	Black	Asian	Hispanic	Mexican American	White	Black	Asian	Hispanic	Mexican American
1988–1994	9.7	10.6	–	–	14.8	8.6	14.5	–	–	13.8
1999–2000	10.9	16.4	–	–	23.5	11.1	21.4	–	–	16.8
2001–2002	15.0	15.5	–	–	22.0	12.7	19.5	–	–	17.0
2003–2004	17.8	16.4	–	–	22.0	14.9	23.8	–	–	16.1
2005–2006	13.4	18.3	–	–	24.3	12.2	24.4	–	–	20.6
2007–2008	15.6	17.3	–	24.5	24.9	14.9	22.8	–	17.3	16.6
2009–2010	16.1	24.3	–	23.4	24.0	11.7	24.3	–	18.9	18.2
2011–2012	12.6	19.9	11.5	24.1	24.2	15.6	20.5	5.6	20.6	21.1
2013–2014	15.9	16.8	12.1	20.6	19.5	14.6	20.9	5.0	22.1	24.2

Source: Fryar, Cheryl D., Margaret D. Carroll, and Cynthia L. Ogden. 2016. "Prevalence of Overweight and Obesity among Children and Adolescents Aged 2–19 Years: United States, 1963–1965 through 2013–2014." National Center for Health Statistics, Table 3. https://www.cdc.gov/nchs/data/hestat/obesity_child_13_14/obesity_child_13_14.pdf. Accessed on April 6, 2017.

Note: –, no data.

Table 5.5   Prevalence of Certain Eating Disorders in the United States

Useful data and statistics about the prevalence of various eating disorders in the United States are limited. Most of the information available on the subject has come from the Centers for Disease Control and Prevention's National Health and Nutrition Examination Survey (NHANES). Prevalence data from various annual NHANES reports include the following:

- Lifetime prevalence (an event that has occurred at least once in a person's lifetime) for anorexia nervosa is 0.6 percent.
- Lifetime prevalence for females is 0.6 percent; for males, 0.3 percent.
- 33.8 percent of those diagnosed with anorexia nervosa are receiving treatment for the disorder.
- Average age of onset for anorexia nervosa is 19 years.
- 12-month prevalence of bulimia nervosa (an event in existence during the past year) is 0.3 percent; lifetime prevalence for the condition is 0.6 percent.
- 12-month prevalence of bulimia nervosa for females is 0.5 percent; for males, 0.1 percent. Lifetime prevalence for females is 1.5 percent; for males, 0.5 percent.
- Average age of onset for bulimia nervosa is 20 years.
- 15.6 percent of those with bulimia nervosa during the last year are receiving treatment; 43.2 percent of those with the condition at least once in their lifetime is 43.2 percent.
- 12-month prevalence of binge eating disorder is 1.2 percent; lifetime prevalence is 2.8 percent.
- 12-month prevalence of binge eating disorder for females is 1.6 percent; for males, 0.8 percent. Lifetime prevalence for females is 3.5 percent; for males, 2.0 percent.
- 28.4 percent of those with binge eating disorder in the last year are receiving treatment; 43.6 percent with lifetime prevalence are receiving treatment.
- Lifetime prevalence of any eating disorder among 13- to 18-year-olds is 2.7 percent. Lifetime prevalence for females in that age group is 3.8 percent; for males, 1.5 percent. Lifetime prevalence for 13- to 14-year-olds is 2.4 percent; for 15- to 16-year-olds, 2.8 percent; for 17- to 18-year-olds, 3.0 percent.

Source: "Eating Disorders." 2016. National Institutes of Mental Health. https://www.nimh.nih.gov/health/topics/eating-disorders/index.shtml. Accessed on June 12, 2017. (See list of statistical data available at end of the article.)

Documents

National Eating Disorders Screening Program (2000)

Probably the most comprehensive research study on eating disorders among school students was conducted under the auspices of the Centers for Disease Control and Prevention in 2000. The study *consisted of a self-administered questionnaire about personal eat-ing habits and attitudes. The following selections summarize the methods used in the study and its primary results. (Omitted refer-ences are indicated by triple asterisks, ***.)*

Methods

The NEDSP Program

NEDSP staff sent out registration information about the pro-gram by direct mail and e-mail to individual membership lists of national professional organizations for school psychologists, nurses, and counselors to invite high schools across the country to enroll in the program. Representatives from high schools then contacted NEDSP to enroll. All participating high schools were provided with a questionnaire to screen for student eat-ing disorders; educational materials for use in classrooms or assemblies; and technical assistance to help staff implement the screening, handle student requests to discuss eating disorders, and make appropriate referrals for evaluation and treatment. NEDSP educational materials included a video and discussion guide, participatory classroom curriculum, and activity guide. All materials were designed to help motivate students to seek help with eating disorder symptoms. Care was taken to design materials that did not glamorize eating disorders or provide unnecessary details about disordered weight control methods. Educational content addressed healthy diet and activity, signs and symptoms to watch out for in friends and family, avail-ability and efficacy of treatment, and the need to seek help for symptoms. In addition, materials offered students guidance on how to talk with a friend or family member who may have an eating disorder ***.

Screening Questionnaire

High schools administered the anonymous, self-report eating disorders screening questionnaire to students in classrooms and assemblies. The survey included the Eating Attitudes Test (EAT-26), a validated eating disorders screening instrument ***. Possible scores on the EAT-26 range from 0 to 78. A score of 20 or above indicates that a person may have an eating disorder and should be evaluated further by a mental health professional. The student screening questionnaire also included items that assessed how often in the past 3 months students had vomited to control their weight, engaged in eating binges, or exercised to lose or control their weight. Each of these behavioral questions was followed by 7 response options: never, less than once per month, 1–3 times per month, once per week, 2–6 times per week, once per day, and more than once per day. The item on vomiting was adapted from the YRBSS ***. The questionnaire included an item on past treatment for eating disorders and items on sex, age, race/ethnicity, height, and weight.

Participants and Sampling Procedure

A total of 270 public, private, and parochial high schools signed up to participate in the screening program, and 152 schools from 34 states completed the screening and educational components of NEDSP. Ninety-eight schools returned more than 35,000 student screening forms for analysis. Because of cost constraints on data entry, a subset of student screening forms were randomly selected for analysis by using a 2-stage, clustered-sampling method. First, 33 schools were randomly sampled from the 98 that returned screening forms, then a random sample of forms was selected from these schools; the number of forms selected from a school was proportional to the number received from that school. Because of a change in protocol at the data entry site, 8 of the 33 schools had all of their surveys entered rather than a proportional random sample; therefore, weighting was used in analyses to adjust for the oversampling of student surveys from these 8 schools. This 2-stage selection procedure resulted in a sample of 5,740 screening forms.

***

Results

The sample included 58% (3,252) girls and 42% (2,315) boys; 3% (189) were African American, 2% (93) American Indian, 2% (134) Asian/Pacific Islander, 5% (303) Latino, 83% (4,629) white, and 4% (219) reported no ethnicity. The mean age was 15.9 (standard deviation 1.0) years. Girls were 3 to 5 times more likely than boys to score at or above the threshold on the EAT-26, to report vomiting to control their weight in the past 3 months, and to have ever been treated for an eating disorder ***.

Among girls, few significant differences were found in eating disorder symptoms across racial/ethnic groups ***. Compared with white girls, Latina girls were less likely and American Indian girls were more likely to score 20 or more on the EAT-26, and African American and American Indian girls were more likely to report exercising more than once per day to control their weight. In contrast, among boys, African American, American Indian, Asian/Pacific Islander, and Latino boys were consistently more symptomatic than were white boys across the range of disordered eating and weight control symptoms and behaviors.

Within symptom subgroups defined by EAT-26 score and binge eating, girls were roughly 3.5 times more likely to report that they had been treated for an eating disorder than were boys with comparable symptom severity ***. Within the symptom subgroup defined by exercising once a day or more often to control weight, girls were almost 8 times more likely than boys to report having been treated for an eating disorder. In contrast, within the subgroup that reported vomiting, no sex difference was observed in the odds of having ever received treatment. In most models, extreme thinness was positively associated with the odds of having been treated for an eating disorder, but age and race/ethnicity were not, controlling for sex and symptom type and severity (data not shown).

Source: Austin, S. Bryn, et al. 2008. "Screening High School Students for Eating Disorders: Results of a National Initiative." *Preventing Chronic Disease.* 5(4): 1–10. https://www.cdc.gov/pcd/issues/2008/oct/pdf/07_0164.pdf.

Frank v. United Airlines (2000)

There is very little case law concerning eating disorder issues. The one area in which such cases might arise—and, to some extent, already have arisen—involves the American with Disabilities Act of 1990 (ADA), as amended. That act prohibits discrimination against an individual because of some physical or mental disability. The act does not itself delineate the specific conditions that are or are not covered by the act, so years of rule-making and litigation have, over time, developed such a list. For individuals and organizations concerned with eating disorders, the argument has long been that conditions such as anorexia, bulimia, and binge eating disorder should be considered to be "disabilities," within the meaning of the ADA and, therefore, covered by its antidiscrimination provisions. One of the early cases to test this argument was Frank v. United Airlines, *in which a group of airline stewardesses sued the airline, arguing that the airline's long-standing weight policies for its employees violated not only the ADA but also the Civil Rights Act of 1946, the Age Discrimination in Employment Act, and the California Fair Employment Act. Essentially they claimed that the airline regulations placed an undue burden on their personal lives, contributing to their weight problems and thus significantly affecting their own quality of life. Both the district court and the Federal Court of Appeals for the Ninth District rejected this argument and ruled in favor of the airline. The major points presented in the court opinion are as follows. (Triple asterisks, ***, indicate the omission of citations and other irrelevant material.)*

The court begins by reviewing the plaintiffs' arguments:

1. From 1980 to 1994, defendant United Airlines, Inc. ("United") required flight attendants to comply with maximum weight requirements based on sex, height and age. Failure to maintain weight below the applicable maximum subjected a flight attendant to various forms of discipline, including suspension without pay and termination. In 1992, plaintiffs filed this action on behalf of a class of female flight attendants to challenge these weight requirements.

2. Plaintiffs contend that by adopting a discriminatory weight policy and enforcing that policy in a discriminatory manner, United discriminated against women and older flight attendants in violation of Title VII of the Civil Rights Act of 1964 ("Title VII"), 42 U.S.C. S 2000e; the Age Discrimination in Employment Act ("ADEA"), 29 U.S.C. SS 621–634; the Americans with Disabilities Act ("ADA"), 42 U.S.C. SS 12101–12213; and the California Fair Employment and Housing Act ("FEHA"), Cal. Gov't Code SS 12900–12996. The district court granted summary judgment for defendant on all of plaintiffs' class and individual claims. ***

3. During the 1960s and early 1970s, the standard practice among large commercial airlines was to hire only women as flight attendants. The airlines required their flight attendants to remain unmarried, to refrain from having children, to meet weight and appearance criteria, and to retire by the age of 35. *** Like other airlines, defendant United had a long-standing practice of requiring female flight attendants to maintain their weight below certain levels. After it began hiring male flight attendants in the wake of Diaz v. Pan Am. World Airways, Inc., 442 F.2d 385 (5th Cir. 1971), United applied maximum weight requirements to both male and female flight attendants. *** Flight attendants—a group comprised of approximately 85% women during the time period relevant to this suit—are the only employees United has ever subjected to maximum weight requirements. United abandoned its weight requirements for flight attendants in 1994.

4. Between 1980 and 1994, United required female flight attendants to weigh between 14 and 25 pounds less than their male colleagues of the same height and age. For example, the maximum weight for a 5' 7", 30-year-old woman was 142 pounds, while a man of the same height and age could weigh up to 161 pounds. A 5' 11", 50-year-old woman could weigh up to 162 pounds, while the limit for a man of

the same height and age was 185 pounds. United's weight table for men during this period was based on a table of desirable weights and heights published by the Metropolitan Life Insurance Company ("MetLife"). The comparable weight table for women was based on a table of maximum weights established by Continental Air Lines ("Continental"). A comparison of United's MetLife-derived limits for men to the Continental derived weight limits for women reveals that United generally limited men to maximum weights that corresponded to large body frames for men on the MetLife charts but generally limited women to maximum weights that corresponded to medium body frames for women on MetLife charts.

5. The thirteen named plaintiffs worked for United as flight attendants while United's 1980–1994 weight policy was in effect. The named plaintiffs attempted to lose weight by various means, including severely restricting their caloric intake, using diuretics, and purging. Ultimately, however, plaintiffs were each disciplined and/or terminated for failing to comply with United's maximum weight requirements. In 1992, plaintiffs filed this employment discrimination action. They sought to represent plaintiff classes of female flight attendants for claims of sex and age discrimination, and they asserted various claims of individual discrimination.

***

The court then deals with aspects of the case other than eating disorders, such as discrimination on the basis of sex (different weight standards for men and women) and age, before focusing on eating disorder issues.

45 We affirm the district court's decision granting summary judgment for United on named plaintiffs' individual claims under the ADA and their corresponding claims under FEHA. The district court correctly concluded that none of the named

plaintiffs presented evidence to make a prima facie case that their eating disorders "substantially limited" a major life activity and were therefore disabilities within the meaning of the ADA. *** A major life activity is a function such as "caring for oneself, performing manual tasks, walking, seeing, hearing, speaking, breathing, learning, and working." *** While eating disorders can substantially limit major life activities, they have not presented evidence that their eating disorders have that effect.

Source: *Leslie Frank, Pat Parnell, Susan Broderick, Carole Kirk, Nichkol Melanson, Sandra Huff, Diane Davis, Sharon Benjamin, Sharron K. Taylor, Bland Lane, Joan Balla Weaver, Donna Durkin, Ellen McCormick v. United Airlines, Inc.,* 216 F.3d 845 (9th Cir. 2000).

H.R. 4310 (2009)

Obesity is generally not regarded for legislative action in the U.S. Congress. From time to time, however, someone will introduce a bill designed to deal with the growing problem of overweight and obesity in the United States. Such was the purpose of H.R. 4310, introduced into the first session of the 111th Congress in December 2009, by Representative Dennis Kuncinich (D-OH). The main features of that bill, which never received consideration by any committee or by the House itself, are provided here. (Triple asterisks, ***, indicate the omission of irrelevant materials.)

A BILL

To amend the Internal Revenue Code of 1986 to protect children's health by denying any deduction for advertising and marketing directed at children to promote the consumption of food at fast food restaurants or of food of poor nutritional quality.

Be it enacted by the Senate and House of Representatives of the United States of America in Congress assembled,

SECTION 1. DENIAL OF DEDUCTION FOR ADVERTISING DIRECTED AT CHILDREN TO PROMOTE THE CONSUMPTION OF FOOD AT FAST FOOD RESTAURANTS OR OF FOOD OF POOR NUTRITIONAL QUALITY.

(a) IN GENERAL.—Part IX of subchapter B of chapter 1 of the Internal Revenue Code of 1986 (relating to items not deductible) is amended by adding at the end the following new section:

"SEC. 280I. DENIAL OF DEDUCTION FOR ADVERTISING DIRECTED AT CHILDREN TO PROMOTE THE CONSUMPTION OF FOOD AT FAST FOOD RESTAURANTS OR OF FOOD OF POOR NUTRITIONAL QUALITY.

"(a) IN GENERAL.—No deduction shall be allowed under this chapter with respect to—

"(1) any advertisement primarily directed at children for purposes of promoting the consumption by children of food from any fast food restaurant or of any food of poor nutritional quality, and

"(2) any of the following which are incurred or provided primarily for purposes described in paragraph (1):

"(A) Travel expenses (including meals and lodging).

"(B) Goods or services of a type generally considered to constitute entertainment, amusement, or recreation or the use of a facility in 4 connection with providing such goods and services.

"(C) Gifts.

"(D) Other promotion expenses.

"(b) FOOD OF POOR NUTRITIONAL QUALITY.—For purposes of this section, the term 'food of poor nutritional quality' means food that is determined by the Secretary (in consultation with the Secretary of Health and Human Services and the Federal Trade Commission) to provide calories primarily through fats or added sugars and to have minimal amounts of vitamins and minerals.

***

The rest of the bill is devoted to "housekeeping" responsibilities associated with the requirements of the bill, if passed.

Source: H.R. 4310. 111th Congress. 1st Session. https://www.congress.gov/111/bills/hr4310/BILLS-111hr4310ih.pdf.

Healthy, Hunger-Free Kids Act of 2010

*The problem of overweight and obesity in the United States, especially among children and adolescents, has prompted the U.S. Congress to consider a number of bills over the past decade to deal with this problem. In most cases, these bills provide funding for programs developed and implemented by the states to carry out programs designed to educate individuals about the problem of obesity and to develop programs for the prevention and treatment of the condition. One of the landmark pieces of legislation was the Healthy, Hunger-Free Kids Act of 2010, whose major provisions are provided here. (Omitted material is indicated by triple asterisks, ***.)*

TITLE II—REDUCING CHILDHOOD OBESITY AND IMPROVING THE DIETS OF CHILDREN

***

Subtitle D—Miscellaneous
SEC. 241. NUTRITION EDUCATION AND OBESITY PREVENTION GRANT PROGRAM.
(a) IN GENERAL.—The Food and Nutrition Act of 2008 (7 U.S.C. 2011 et seq.) is amended by adding at the end the following:
"SEC. 28. NUTRITION EDUCATION AND OBESITY PREVENTION GRANT PROGRAM.

Section (a) continues with a definition of terms used in the bill.

***

"(b) PROGRAMS.—Consistent with the terms and conditions of grants awarded under this section, State agencies may implement a nutrition education and obesity prevention program for eligible individuals that promotes healthy food choices consistent with the most recent Dietary Guidelines for Americans published under section 301 of the National Nutrition Monitoring and Related Research Act of 1990 (7 U.S.C. 5341).

"(c) DELIVERY OF NUTRITION EDUCATION AND OBESITY PREVENTION SERVICES.—

"(1) IN GENERAL.—State agencies may deliver nutrition education and obesity prevention services under a program described in subsection (b)—

"(A) directly to eligible individuals; or

"(B) through agreements with other State or local agencies or community organizations.

"(2) NUTRITION EDUCATION STATE PLANS.—

"(A) IN GENERAL.—A State agency that elects to provide nutrition education and obesity prevention services under this subsection shall submit to the Secretary for approval a nutrition education State plan.

"(B) REQUIREMENTS.—Except as provided in subparagraph (C), a nutrition education State plan shall—

"(i) identify the uses of the funding for local projects;

"(ii) ensure that the interventions are appropriate for eligible individuals who are members of low-income populations by recognizing the constrained resources, and the potential eligibility for Federal food assistance programs, of members of those populations; and "(iii) conform to standards established by the Secretary through regulations, guidance, or grant award documents.

***

"(3) USE OF FUNDS.—

"(A) IN GENERAL.—A State agency may use funds provided under this section for any evidence-based allowable use of funds identified by the Administrator of the Food and Nutrition Service of the Department of Agriculture in consultation with the Director of the Centers for Disease Control and Prevention of the Department of Health and Human Services, including—

"(i) individual and group-based nutrition education, health promotion, and intervention strategies;

"(ii) comprehensive, multilevel interventions at multiple complementary organizational and institutional levels; and

"(iii) community and public health approaches to improve nutrition.

"(B) CONSULTATION.—In identifying allowable uses of funds under subparagraph (A) and in seeking to strengthen delivery, oversight, and evaluation of nutrition education, the Administrator of the Food and Nutrition Service shall consult with the Director of the Centers for Disease Control and Prevention and outside stakeholders and experts, including—

"(i) representatives of the academic and research communities;

"(ii) nutrition education practitioners;

"(iii) representatives of State and local governments; and

"(iv) community organizations that serve lowincome populations.

***

SEC. 244. RESEARCH ON STRATEGIES TO PROMOTE THE SELECTION AND CONSUMPTION OF HEALTHY FOODS.

(a) IN GENERAL.—The Secretary, in consultation with the Secretary of Health and Human Services, shall establish a research, demonstration, and technical assistance program to promote healthy eating and reduce the prevalence of obesity, among all population groups but especially among children, by applying the principles and insights of behavioral economics research in schools, child care programs, and other settings.

(b) PRIORITIES.—The Secretary shall—

1. identify and assess the impacts of specific presentation, placement, and other strategies for structuring choices on selection and consumption of healthful foods in a variety of settings, consistent with the most recent version of the Dietary Guidelines for Americans published under section 301 of the National Nutrition Monitoring and Related Research Act of 1990 (7 U.S.C. 5341);

2. demonstrate and rigorously evaluate behavioral economics-related interventions that hold promise to improve diets and promote health, including through demonstration projects that may include evaluation of the use of portion size, labeling, convenience, and other strategies to encourage healthy choices; and

3. encourage adoption of the most effective strategies through outreach and technical assistance.

Source: PUBLIC LAW 111–296—DEC. 13, 2010 124 STAT. 3183. https://www.fns.usda.gov/sites/default/files/PL_111-296.pdf.

Child Performer Advisory Board to Prevent Eating Disorders. State of New York (2010)

Regardless of efforts to enact laws dealing with eating disorders at the federal level, a number of states have adopted their own laws of one kind or another to deal with this issue. In 2010, the state legislature of New York adopted new regulations for the employment of minors in the entertainment business (including the modeling business) that would require their learning about the problems of eating disorders. The law had the following provisions.

1. The commissioner, in consultation with the commissioner of health and the commissioner of mental health, shall establish a child performer advisory board for the purpose of recommending guidelines for the employment of child performers and models under the age of eighteen and preventing eating disorders such as anorexia nervosa and bulimia nervosa amongst such persons. The advisory board shall consist of at least sixteen but no more than twenty members appointed by the commissioner, and shall include: representatives of professional organizations or unions representing child performers or models; employers representing child performers or models; physicians, nutritionists and mental health professionals with demonstrated expertise in treating patients with eating disorders; at least one representative from each of the comprehensive care centers for eating disorders established pursuant to article twenty-seven-J of the public health law; advocacy organizations working to prevent and treat eating disorders; and other members deemed necessary by the commissioner. In addition, the commissioner of health and the commissioner of mental health, or their designees, shall serve on the advisory board. The members of the advisory board shall receive no compensation for their services but shall be reimbursed their actual and necessary expenses incurred in the performance of their duties.

2. The advisory board is authorized to develop recommendations to the commissioner establishing guidelines relating to the employment of child performers and models under the

age of eighteen for purposes of preventing and accessing treatment for eating disorders such as anorexia nervosa and bulimia nervosa amongst such child performers and models. When developing such guidelines, the advisory board shall consider (a) body mass index standards or weight and height standards, (b) employment restrictions for persons diagnosed with or suspected of having an eating disorder, (c) requiring medical or mental health screenings, by medical or mental health professionals with demonstrated expertise in the diagnosis and treatment of eating disorders, for persons suspected of having an eating disorder, and (d) requiring referrals for treatment of eating disorders.

3. The advisory board shall further develop recommendations for educational and informational materials for such child performers and models, their parents and/or guardians and their employers regarding awareness and recognition of eating disorders, and referral and treatment information of eating disorders such as anorexia nervosa and bulimia nervosa.

4. The commissioner shall consider the recommendations developed by the advisory board, which include employment guidelines and the development of educational and informational materials pursuant to this section, when adopting, promulgating, amending and rescinding the rules and regulations necessary to carry out the provisions of this section. The advisory board shall report to the commissioner regarding its recommendations, including the guidelines, programs and findings developed pursuant to this section.

Source: Article 4-A. Employment and Education of Child Performers. State of New York Labor Code. https://labor.ny.gov/workerprotection/laborstandards/secure/child_index.shtm.

Harlick v. Blue Shield of California (2011)

A second, more recent, field of case law (see Frank v. United Airlines, *earlier) involves insurance coverage for eating disorder* *treatments. Health insurance policies cover the cost of treatment for a large number of physical and mental disorders, ranging from cancer to schizophrenia. The specific provisions—the list of disorders covered and the extent of coverage—vary from company to company. In the case cited here, the plaintiff, Jeanene Harlick, was denied coverage for a period of intensive care for her anorexia by her insurance provider, Blue Shield of California. Essentially the company argued that, while it did cover some of Harlick's initial costs for treatment of anorexia, it was not required by her policy to cover the extensive stay in a treatment facility that then ensued. Harlick responded by insisting that the policy did cover all the necessary care for her disorder and that, in any case, the state of California's Mental Health Parity Act required Blue Cross to provide this coverage, no matter the possible specific wording of her own contract. The case was quite complicated because both the insurer and the state appeared to have taken differing positions on these arguments over time. In any case, the court eventually ruled that Blue Cross was correct in its claim that Harlick's condition was not covered by the policy. But it also ruled that her claim was covered by provisions of the Mental Health Parity Act, which in and of itself required that Blue Cross cover the needed treatment. The main elements of the court's decision are as follows. (Omitted citations are indicated by triple asterisks, ***.)*

I. Background

A. Harlick's Treatment at Castlewood

Jeanene Harlick, who is now 37 years old, has suffered from anorexia for more than twenty years. In early 2006, when she was a clerk at the Pacific Construction & Manufacturing Company, she relapsed and began undergoing intensive outpatient treatment. She was then enrolled in the company's health insurance plan through Blue Shield ("the Plan"), which paid for the treatment.

In March 2006, Harlick's doctors told her that she needed a higher level of care than the intensive outpatient treatment then being provided. Blue Shield employees told Harlick on the telephone that residential treatment was not covered under her Plan, but that partial or inpatient (full-time) hospitalization would be covered if Blue Shield determined that it was medically necessary. Blue Shield employees gave Harlick the names of several facilities where such treatment might be covered. Harlick and her doctors ultimately determined that none of the in-network facilities suggested by Blue Shield could provide effective treatment, so she registered at Castlewood Treatment Center, a residential treatment facility in Missouri that specializes in eating disorders. When Harlick entered Castlewood, she was at 65% of her ideal body weight. When she had been there less than a month, a feeding tube was inserted because her "caloric level needed to gain weight was so high." Harlick stayed at Castlewood from April 17, 2006 to January 31, 2007.

***

C. Blue Shield's Coverage Decision

Blue Shield paid for the first eleven days of Harlick's treatment at Castlewood, but then refused to pay for the rest of her treatment. Blue Shield conducted several internal reviews of Harlick's claim, and Blue Shield employees engaged in extensive correspondence with Harlick and her mother, Robin Watson, about her claim.

On September 20, 2006, Blue Shield employee Bruce Berg reviewed Harlick's record and recommended denying the claim ***

On December 8, 2006, Blue Shield employee David Battin reviewed the claim in another internal document. Battin concluded that "[t]he principal reason" for the denial was that Harlick's plan did not cover residential care. ***

On January 19, 2007, Blue Shield employee Carroll Cederberg reviewed the claim in another internal document. Cederberg again concluded that residential care was not a covered benefit under Harlick's Plan.

On March 27, 2007, David Battin reviewed the claim again in another internal document. He concluded:

> The principal reason [for the denial] is that these services are not a covered benefit. As per your health plan's Evidence of Coverage (EOC); all inpatient psychiatric hospital care must be prior authorized by the Mental Health Services Administrator (MHSA), except for emergency care. Since you specifically traveled to Missouri to be admitted to this particular facility, this would not be considered as an emergency admission. You also had amble [*sic*] time to contact MHSA for authorization prior to your admission. In addition; [*sic*] residential care (room and board) is not a covered benefit. During the dates of service 4/28/06 to 8/25/06 the medical necessity of being treated as an inpatient was not established, you could have been treated as an outpatient. Since your EOC does not cover room and board, the facility fees for your residential treatment . . . are not a covered benefit.

***

III. Discussion
A. Plan Coverage of Residential Care
For the reasons that follow, we conclude that Harlick's Plan does not itself provide coverage for her residential care at Castlewood.

***

B. Mental Health Parity Act
For the reasons that follow, we conclude that the Mental Health Parity Act requires that a plan within the scope of the Act provide all "medically necessary treatment" for "severe mental illnesses," and that Harlick's residential care at Castlewood was medically necessary.

1. Overview of the Act

[9] The California Mental Health Parity Act ("Parity Act" or "Act") was enacted in 1999. In enacting the statute, the California legislature found that "[m]ost private health insurance policies provide coverage for mental illness at levels far below coverage for other physical illnesses." *** The legislature further found that coverage limitations had resulted in inadequate treatment of mental illnesses, causing "relapse and untold suffering" for people with treatable mental illnesses, as well as increases in homelessness, increases in crime, and significant demands on the state budget. ***

To combat this disparity, the Parity Act provides, in pertinent part:

(a) Every health care service plan contract issued, amended, or renewed on or after July 1, 2000, that provides hospital, medical, or surgical coverage shall provide coverage for the diagnosis and medically necessary treatment of severe mental illnesses of a person of any age . . . under the same terms and conditions applied to other medical conditions as specified in subdivision (c).

(b) These benefits shall include the following:

    (1) Outpatient services.

    (2) Inpatient hospital services.

    (3) Partial hospital services.

    (4) Prescription drugs, if the plan contract includes coverage for prescription drugs.

(c) The terms and conditions applied to the benefits required by this section, that shall be applied equally to all benefits under the plan contract, shall include, but not be limited to, the following:

    (1) Maximum lifetime benefits.

    (2) Copayments.

    (3) Individual and family deductibles.

(d) For the purposes of this section, "severe mental illnesses" shall include:

. . . .

(8) Anorexia nervosa

***

c. Summary

[16] We therefore conclude that the most reasonable interpretation of the Parity Act and its implementing regulation is that plans within the scope of the Act must provide coverage of all "medically necessary treatment" for the nine enumerated "severe mental illnesses" under the same financial terms as those applied to physical illnesses.

***

C. Medical Necessity in Harlick's Case

[17] The remaining question is whether Harlick's residential care at Castlewood was medically necessary. ***

Conclusion

[21] Harlick's Plan does not itself require that Blue Shield pay for residential care at Castlewood for her anorexia nervosa. However, California's Mental Health Parity Act provides that Blue Shield "shall provide coverage for the diagnosis and medically necessary treatment" of "severe mental illnesses," including anorexia nervosa. Blue Shield is foreclosed from asserting that Harlick's residential care at Castlewood was not medically necessary. We therefore conclude that Blue Shield is obligated under the Parity Act to pay for Harlick's residential care at Castlewood, subject to the same financial terms and conditions it imposes on coverage for physical illnesses.

Source: *United States Court of Appeals for the Ninth Circuit. Jeanene Harlick, Plaintiff-appellant, v. Blue Shield of*

California, Defendant-appellee. https://law.justia.com/cases/
federal/appellate-courts/ca9/10-15595/10-15595-2012-06-
04.html.

Educating to Prevent Eating Disorders Act of 2015

*In December 2015, Representative Renee Elmers (R-NC) introduced
legislation to provide federal funding for educational programs on
eating disorders. The bill amended the Public Health Service Act of
1944 to pay for educational programs for teachers and parents on
the dangers of eating disorders. Salient portions of the bill, which
was not acted on by the House of Representatives, are provided here.
(Triple asterisks, ***, indicate the omission of a portion of the bill.)*

A BILL

To amend the Public Health Service Act to establish a pilot
program to test the impact of early intervention on the prevention, management, and course of eating disorders.

***

"(a) IN GENERAL.—The Secretary, through the Director of
the Agency for Healthcare Research and Quality, may establish
a pilot program, for a period of three consecutive school years,
to test the impact of providing students in eligible schools with
interventions to prevent, identify, intervene, and manage eating disorders.
    "(b) GRANTS.—
    "(1) IN GENERAL.—Under such pilot program, the Secre-
tary shall award grants to eligible schools. Each such grant shall
be for the period of the pilot program.
    "(2) USES.—Each eligible school receiving a grant under
the pilot program shall use such grant to—

"(A) develop best practices, in accordance, as appropriate, with
        input from research experts in the eating disorders field, for
        eligible health care providers to assess and recognize stu-
        dents with eating disorders and to respond appropriately;

"(B) hire an eligible health care provider to—

"(i) in accordance with the best practices developed pursuant to subparagraph (A), assess and recognize whether students in grades 6 through 8 attending such school have eating disorders and respond appropriately to individuals with eating disorders among students attending such school, including by providing counsel and by referral;

"(ii) provide educational information and seminars, developed in partnership with research experts in the field of eating disorders, to teachers at such school and parents of students attending such school to assist such teachers and parents in recognizing the symptoms of eating disorders and understanding how to seek help and intervention; and

"(iii) otherwise serve as a full-time health care provider for such school.

***

Remaining sections of the bill define institutions that can be considered "eligible schools," "eligible health-care providers," and reports to the Congress required of progress as a result of the actions described in the bill.

Source: HR. 4153. 114th Congress. 1st Session. https://www .congress.gov/114/bills/hr4153/BILLS-114hr4153ih.pdf.

Stop Obesity in Schools Act of 2015

Since the passage of the Healthy, Hunger-Free Kids Act of 2010 (see earlier), other bills have been submitted in the U.S. Congress designed to reduce the rate of childhood obesity in the nation. Thus far, none has passed. The Stop Obesity in Schools Act of 2015 illustrates the type of recommendations that at least some members of Congress are recommending for dealing with the obesity problem. (Triple asterisks, ***, indicate the omission of text.)

Section 1 assigns a title to this act.

Section 1 summarizes the Congress's findings about childhood obesity.

SEC. 3. NATIONAL STRATEGY TO REDUCE CHILD-HOOD OBESITY.

The Secretary of Health and Human Services, in cooperation with State, local, and tribal governments, Federal agencies, local educational agencies, health care providers, the research community, and the private sector, shall develop a national strategy to reduce childhood obesity in the United States. Such strategy shall—

1. provide for the reduction of childhood obesity rates by 10 percent by the year 2020;

2. address both short- and long-term solutions to reducing the rates of childhood obesity in the United States;

3. identify how the Federal Government can work effectively with State, local, and tribal governments, local educational agencies, health care providers, the research community, the private sector, and other entities as necessary to implement the strategy; and

4. include measures to identify and overcome all obstacles to achieving the goal of reducing childhood obesity in the United States.

Section 4 provides information on grants to carry out obesity programs in the states.

***

SEC. 5. EVALUATION OF PROGRAMS FOR THE PREVENTION OF OBESITY IN CHILDREN AND ADOLESCENTS.

(a) IN GENERAL.—For the purpose described in subsection (b), the Director shall (directly or through grants or contracts awarded to public or nonprofit private entities) arrange for the evaluation of a wide variety of existing programs designed in whole or in part to prevent obesity in children and adolescents, including programs that do not receive grants from the Federal Government for operation.

(b) PURPOSE.—The purpose of the evaluation under this section shall be to determine the following:

1. The effectiveness of programs in reducing obesity in children and adolescents.
2. The factors contributing to the effectiveness of the programs.
3. The feasibility of replicating the programs in other locations.

More information on grants follows.

***

SEC. 6. HEALTHY LIVING AND WELLNESS COORDINATING COUNCILS.

(a) GRANTS.—The Director shall make grants on a competitive basis to State, local, or tribal governments, and consortia of such governments, to reduce childhood obesity through—

1. establishing or expanding healthy living and wellness coordinating councils; and
2. supporting regional workshops.

(b) USES OF FUNDS.—As a condition on the receipt of a grant under this section, an entity shall agree to use the grant to carry out one or more of the following:

1. Establishing a healthy living and wellness coordinating council.
2. Expanding the activities of a healthy living and wellness coordinating council, including by implementing State-based

or regionwide activities that will reduce the rates of childhood obesity.

3. Supporting regional workshops designed to permit educators, administrators, health care providers, and other relevant parties to share successful research-based strategies for increasing healthy living and reducing obesity in elementary and secondary schools.

The remaining pages of the act deal with "housekeeping" issues and definitions used in the bill.

Source: H.R. 3772. 114th Congress. 1st Session. https://www .congress.gov/114/bills/hr3772/BILLS-114hr3772ih.pdf.

Having Body Image Issues (2015)

Girlshealth.gov is a website created by the Office of Women's Health of the U.S. Department of Health and Human Services in 2002. It is intended to provide advice and resources for young women about a variety of health topics, eating disorders being one of them. The following extract from the website deals with one important aspect of eating disorders, one's own body image. (The presence of three asterisks, ***, indicates material on the website that has been omitted for this selection.)

Do you wish you could lose weight, get taller, or develop faster? It's pretty common to worry a little about how your body looks, especially when it's changing. You can learn about body image and ways to take control of yours.

***

What is body image?

Body image is how you think and feel about your body. It includes whether you think you look good to other people.

Body image is affected by a lot of things, including messages you get from your friends, family, and the world around you.

Images we see in the media definitely affect our body image even though a lot of media images are changed or aren't realistic.

Why does body image matter? Your body image can affect how you feel about yourself overall. For example, if you are unhappy with your looks, your self-esteem may start to go down. Sometimes, having body image issues or low self-esteem may lead to depression, eating disorders, or obesity.

How can I deal with body image issues?

Everyone has something they would like to change about their bodies. But you'll be happier if you focus on the things you like about your body—and your whole self. Need some help? Check out some tips:

- List your great traits. If you start to criticize your body, tell yourself to stop. Instead, think about what you like about yourself, both inside and out. The "What's unique about me?" log can get you started.

- Know your power. Hey, your body is not just a place to hang your clothes! It can do some truly amazing things. Focus on how strong and healthy your body can be.

- Treat your body well. Eat right, sleep tight, and get moving. You'll look and feel your best—and you'll be pretty proud of yourself too.

- Give your body a treat. Take a nice bubble bath, do some stretching, or just curl up on a comfy couch. Do something soothing.

- Mind your media. Try not to let models and actresses affect how you think you should look. They get lots of help from makeup artists, personal trainers, and photo fixers. And advertisers often use a focus on thinness to get people to buy stuff. Don't let them mess with your mind!

- Let yourself shine. A lot of how we look comes from how we carry ourselves. Feeling proud, walking tall, and smiling big can boost your beauty—and your mood.

- Find fab friends. Your best bet is to hang out with people who accept you for you! And work with your friends to support each other.

If you can't seem to accept how you look, talk to an adult you trust. You can get help feeling better about your body.

***

Stressing about body changes

During puberty and your teen years, your body changes a lot. All those changes can be hard to handle. They might make you worry about what other people think of how you look and about whether your body is normal. If you have these kinds of concerns, you are not alone.

Here are some common thoughts about changing bodies.

- Why am I taller than most of the boys my age?
- Why haven't I grown?
- Am I too skinny?
- Am I too fat?
- Will others like me now [*sic*] that I am changing?
- Are my breasts too small?
- Are my breasts too large?
- Why do I have acne?
- Do my clothes look right on my body?
- Are my hips getting bigger?

If you are stressed about your body, you may feel better if you understand why you are changing so fast—or not changing as fast as your friends.

During puberty, you get taller and see other changes in your body, such as wider hips and thighs. Your body will also start to have more fat compared to muscle than before. Each young woman changes at her own pace, and all of these changes are normal.

Want to know more about how your body and mind may be changing? You can read all about puberty. You also can work on feeling good about your body while it's changing.

What are serious body image problems?

If how your body looks bothers you a lot and you can't stop thinking about it, you could have body dysmorphic disorder, or BDD.

People with BDD think they look ugly even if they have a small flaw or none at all. They may spend many hours a day looking at flaws and trying to hide them. They also may ask friends to reassure them about their looks or want to have a lot of cosmetic surgery. If you or a friend may have BDD, talk to an adult you trust, such as a parent or guardian, school counselor, teacher, doctor, or nurse. BDD is an illness, and you can get help.

Source: "Having Body Image Issues." 2015. Girlshealth.gov. https://www.girlshealth.gov/feelings/bodyimage/index.html.

Tennessee School Health Screening Guidelines (2015)

One of the recommendations that has been made for identifying, preventing, and treating eating disorders among students is called the school screening option. Most schools now routinely screen students at one or another grade levels for possible physical problems such as poor vision or hearing. (A screening test is one that is given to all members of a population, whether or not they are thought to be at risk for a physical or mental problem.) Some experts have suggested that tests for eating disorders might be included among regular school screenings, and some states have moved at least in part to the adoption of such programs. The following selection is taken from a booklet provided by the Tennessee Department of Health and the Tennessee Department of Education to help educators and parents understand the importance of being alert for possible eating disorders. The state has not yet adopted a plan for formally including such screening yet.

G.7 Eating Disorders/Malnutrition

Although considered to be mental health disorders, eating disorders are remarkable for their association with nutrition-related problems. In anorexia nervosa, nutrition-related problems include refusal to maintain a minimally healthy body weight (e.g., 85% of that expected), dramatic weight loss, fear of gaining weight even though underweight, preoccupation with food, and abnormal food consumption patterns. Anorexia nervosa is 10 times more common in females, especially just after onset of puberty, peaking at ages 12–13 years. Bulimia nervosa is an eating disorder with food addiction as the primary coping mechanism. In bulimia nervosa, problems include recurrent episodes of binge eating, a sense of lack of control over eating, and compensatory behavior after binge eating to prevent weight gain (e.g., self-induced vomiting, abuse of laxatives or diuretics, fasting). Body weight is often normal or slightly above normal.

Students identified to be at risk for malnutrition or failure-to-thrive or who are suspected to have eating disorders should be referred to a primary care provider for in-depth medical assessment. These nutrition-related conditions must be addressed cautiously and expediently. Aside from psychological disturbances, eating disorders can lead to serious electrolyte imbalances and dehydration. Long-term effects include osteoporosis. Death can occur in extreme cases. Because of the serious nature of these potential conditions, it is imperative that school health personnel communicate observations and concerns directly to the parent/guardian. Effective treatment for eating disorders involves medical and psychological treatment, nutritional counseling, and family and school support. Keep in mind that a diagnosis of an eating disorder can be made only by a physician or an appropriate health care provider.

Source: "Tennessee School Health Screening Guidelines." 2015. Tennessee Department of Health and Tennessee Department

of Education. https://www.tn.gov/content/dam/tn/education/
csh/csh_school_health_screening_guidelines.pdf.

State of Missouri. Senate Bill No. 145 (2015)

One of the recommendations made by experts in the field of eating disorders is that testing and treatment be made more readily available by requiring insurance companies to include payment for such services in their contracts. The first state to adopt this policy was Missouri, where in 2015, Senate Bill 145 was passed by the legislature and signed by Governor Jay Nixon. Relevant portions of that bill are included here.

Section A. Chapter 376, RSMo, is amended by adding thereto one new section, to be known as section 376.845, to read as follows:

[Part (1) of the bill then defines all terms used in the bill, such as "eating disorder," "health benefit plan," "health carrier," and "health care."]

2. In accordance with the provisions of section 376.1550, all 52 health benefit plans that are delivered, issued for delivery, continued or renewed on or after January 1, 2017, if written inside the state of Missouri, or written outside the state of Missouri but covering Missouri residents, shall provide coverage for the diagnosis and treatment of eating disorders as required in section 376.1550.

3. Coverage provided under this section is limited to medically necessary treatment that is provided by a licensed treating physician, psychiatrist, psychologist, professional counselor, clinical social worker, or licensed marital and family therapist pursuant to the powers granted under such licensed physician's, psychiatrist's, psychologist's, professional counselor's, clinical social worker's, or licensed marital and family therapist's license and acting within their applicable scope of coverage, in accordance with a treatment plan.

4. The treatment plan, upon request by the health benefit plan or health carrier, shall include all elements necessary for the

health benefit plan or health carrier to pay claims. Such elements include, but are not limited to, a diagnosis, proposed treatment by type, frequency and duration of treatment, and goals.

5. Coverage of the treatment of eating disorders may be subject to other general exclusions and limitations of the contract or benefit plan not in conflict with the provisions of this section, such as coordination of benefits, and utilization review of health care services, which includes reviews of medical necessity and care management. Medical necessity determinations and care management for the treatment of eating disorders shall consider the overall medical and mental health needs of the individual with an eating disorder, shall not be based solely on weight, and shall take into consideration the most recent Practice Guideline for the Treatment of Patients with Eating Disorders adopted by the American Psychiatric Association in addition to current standards based upon the medical literature generally recognized as authoritative in the medical community.

Source: Senate Bill No. 45. 98th General Assembly. 2015. State of Missouri. http://www.senate.mo.gov/15info/pdf-bill/tat/SB145.pdf.

21st Century Cures Act (2016)

The 21st Century Cures Act was the first piece of federal legislation adopted by both houses of the U.S. Congress. The act provided $6.3 billion, most of which went to the National Institutes of Health, for a variety of programs designed to improve mental health care in the United States. After passage of the act, NBC News called the action "the most significant mental health reform bill in decades" (Morris 2017). One component of the final act was a bill passed earlier by the House of Representatives called the Helping Families in Mental Health Crisis Act of 2016, which itself contained two sections dealing specifically with eating disorders. The relevant parts of the 21st Century

Cures Act are included here. (Omitted sections are indicated by triple asterisks, ***.)

An Act

To accelerate the discovery, development, and delivery of 21st century cures, and for other purposes.

***

SEC. 13005. INFORMATION AND AWARENESS ON EATING DISORDERS.

(a) INFORMATION.—The Secretary of Health and Human Services, acting through the Director of the Office on Women's Health, may—

1. update information, related fact sheets, and resource lists related to eating disorders that are available on the public Internet website of the National Women's Health Information Center sponsored by the Office on Women's Health, to include—

    (A) updated findings and current research related to eating disorders, as appropriate; and

    (B) information about eating disorders, including information related to males and females;

2. incorporate, as appropriate, and in coordination with the Secretary of Education, information from publicly available resources into appropriate obesity prevention programs developed by the Office on Women's Health; and

3. make publicly available (through a public Internet website or other method) information, related fact sheets, and resource lists, as updated under paragraph (1), and the information incorporated into appropriate obesity prevention programs under paragraph (2).

(b) AWARENESS.—The Secretary of Health and Human Services may advance public awareness on—

1. the types of eating disorders;
2. the seriousness of eating disorders, including prevalence, co-morbidities, and physical and mental health consequences;
3 methods to identify, intervene, refer for treatment, and prevent behaviors that may lead to the development of eating disorders;
4. discrimination and bullying based on body size;
5. the effects of media on self-esteem and body image; and
6. the signs and symptoms of eating disorders.

SEC. 13006. EDUCATION AND TRAINING ON EATING DISORDERS.

The Secretary of Health and Human Services may facilitate the identification of model programs and materials for educating and training health professionals in effective strategies to—

1. identify individuals with eating disorders;
2. provide early intervention services for individuals with eating disorders;
3. refer patients with eating disorders for appropriate treatment;
4. prevent the development of eating disorders; and
5. provide appropriate treatment services for individuals with eating disorders.

Reference

Morris, Kurt. 2017. "Could the Author of the New Health Bill Be Any More Hypocritical?" Tonic. https://tonic .vice.com/en_us/article/gy5jqy/could-the-author-of-the-healthcare-bill-be-any-more-hypocritical. Accessed on November 28, 2018.

Source: H.R. 34. 114th Congress. Second Session. https://www.gpo.gov/fdsys/pkg/BILLS-114hr34enr/pdf/BILLS-114hr34enr.pdf.

Assembly Bill No. 2539. State of California (2016)

For many observers, possibly the most serious factor responsible for the nation's eating disorder problem is the "ideal" standard established by corporations, mass media, professional sporting operations, and similar agencies with an impact on public standards for weight and appearance. In 2015, California assemblyman Marc Levine filed legislation to institute controls over modeling agencies designed to deal with this issue. The bill was the first of its kind in the United States. The bill was not passed in 2016 but was reintroduced in 2017 and 2018. As of late 2018, no action had been taken on the bill. (The bill has been revised since its introduction, and the excerpt here contains only its most recent version. Omissions in the text provided here are indicated by triple asterisks, ***.)

An act to add Chapter 6 (commencing with Section 1707) to Part 6 of Division 2 of the Labor Code, relating to modeling agencies.

***

1707. The Legislature finds and declares all of the following:

(a) __Professional fashion models face pervasive and hazardous occupational demands to maintain extreme and unhealthy thinness. These occupational pressures create a dangerous work environment. Models experience a substantially elevated risk of eating disorders and other severe health problems associated with starvation.

(b) __The majority of models enter the industry as minors, making them especially vulnerable to mistreatment and to the physical and psychological damage caused by eating disorders. Women working as professional fashion models are more likely to have a diagnosis of anorexia nervosa, dangerously low body mass index, and amenorrhea, which is a serious medical indicator of hormonal dysregulation that can have negative health consequences for life.

(c) __As with all workers, professional fashion models are entitled to safe working conditions. The time, place, and means of the services provided by professional models are typically controlled by the company paying their compensation. ***

Many models, including minors, are wrongly treated as independent contractors *** and currently do not receive workplace protections. Clarifying their classification as employees of the companies paying their compensation will enhance *** workplace protections.

(d) __The impact of the fashion industry on health reaches far beyond the hazardous occupational conditions that professional 20 models endure. Through its dominant presence in the mass media and pervasive influence on setting cultural standards for apparel, particularly for girls and young women, the fashion industry helps to define, transmit, and reinforce an unrealistic standard of thinness, a well-documented risk factor for eating disorders.

(e) __Scientific research has shown that viewing media images of extremely thin models leads to body dissatisfaction in adolescent girls and young women, especially those who already have heightened vulnerability to eating disorders. In addition, scientific studies have shown that body dissatisfaction in adolescence is a strong indicator that a young person may develop an eating disorder.

(f) __Improving working conditions to reduce excessive thinness among professional models is likely to lead to healthier images of models' weight. This change in media portrayals of models' weight may help to achieve a larger societal value in making media images more healthful and less damaging to girls' and young women's body image, ultimately reducing their risk for eating disorders.

Section 1707.1 provides definitions for all important terms used in the bill.

1707.3. A person shall not engage in or carry on the occupation of a modeling agency without first procuring a license *** under Chapter 4 (commencing with Section 1700) ***

Section 1707.4 is deleted.

1707.5. (a)__The Occupational Safety and Health Standards Board *** shall, no later than December 1, 2017, and in consultation with accredited specialists in the prevention and treatment of eating disorders, adopt an occupational safety and health standard for models, with an operative date of September 1, 2018, to be fully complied with by December 31, 2018. The standard shall apply to services provided in California by models under this chapter and Chapter 4 (commencing with Section 1700). The Occupational Safety and Health Standards Board may update these standards from time to time as it deems necessary.

***

(b)__The *** standard shall *** address issues 30 including, but not limited to, all of the following:

1. __Protection of the model's rights to health care privacy under the Health Insurance Portability and Accountability Act of 1996 (Public Law 104-191) and all other provisions of law.

2. __Workplace safety, especially for minors, including protection from sexual exploitation and sexual predators.

3. __Prevention and treatment of eating disorders.

Source: Assembly Bill No. 2539. California State Legislature. http://www.leginfo.ca.gov/pub/15-16/bill/asm/ab_2501-2550/ab_2539_bill_20160330_amended_asm_v98.pdf.

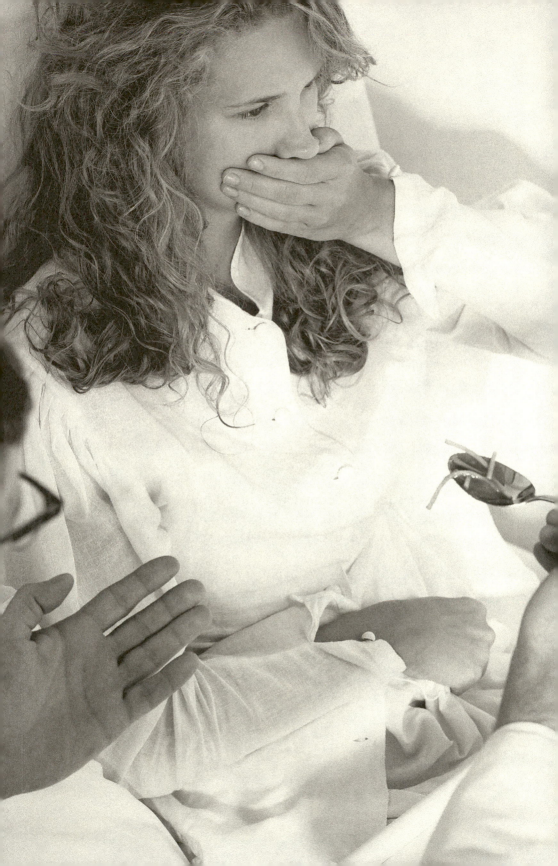

Introduction

Information about the causes, prevention, and treatment of eating disorders is of interest to many young adults, parents, specialists in the field, and the layperson. A great deal has been written in books, articles, and reports and on the Internet about these issues. This chapter provides a sample of some of these print and electronic resources. Some overlap or duplication exists when a print article also appears on the Internet or vice versa. In such cases, both sources are listed in this bibliography.

Books

Adan, Roger A. H., and Walter H. Kaye, eds. 2013. *Behavioral Neurobiology of Eating Disorders*. Berlin: Springer.

> This collection of essays provides a good, if technical, introduction to recent research on the neurobiological basis of eating disorder. Chapters discuss topics such as neurocircuitry of eating disorders, the role of serotonin and dopamine, the genetics of eating disorders, animal models in eating disorders, and translating experimental neuroscience into treatment of eating disorders.

A doctor counsels a young anorexic hospital patient as she rejects food. (Katarzyna Bialasiewicz/Dreamstime.com)

American Psychiatric Association. 2013. *Diagnostic and Statistical Manual of Mental Disorders, Fifth Edition*. Arlington, VA: American Psychiatric Association.

>   This book is the ultimate guide to the identification and diagnosis of mental disorders. Definitions, characteristics, and possible treatment considered from the standpoint of the psychiatric profession are all available in this text in pages 361–395.

Arnold, Carrie. 2013. *Decoding Anorexia: How Breakthroughs in Science Offer Hope for Eating Disorders*. London: Routledge.

>   The author provides a review of the role of anorexia in human history before outlining some of the most recent discoveries in science relating to the cause, progress, prevention, and treatment of anorexia.

Brewerton, Timothy D., and Amy Baker Dennis. 2014. *Eating Disorders, Addictions and Substance Use Disorders: Research, Clinical and Treatment Perspectives*. Berlin; Heidelberg: Springer.

>   This book summarizes current information about the correlates and comorbidities of eating disorders, with chapters on "Are Eating Disorders Addictions?," "Genetic Vulnerability to Eating Disorders and Substance Abuse Disorders," "Bariatric Surgery and Substance Use Disorders, Eating Disorders, and Other Impulse Control Disorders," "Prevention of Eating Disorders and Substance Misuse in Adolescence," and "Medical Complications of Eating Disorders, Substance Use Disorders, and Addictions."

Brownell, Kelly D., and B. Timothy Walsh. 2017. *Eating Disorders and Obesity: A Comprehensive Handbook*, 3rd ed. New York: The Guilford Press.

>   This book includes more than 100 chapters on a vast array of issues related to eating disorders and obesity. It is a treasure chest of the most recent information available on nearly every aspect of the conditions.

Brumberg, Joan Jacobs. 2001. *Fasting Girls: The History of Anorexia Nervosa*. New York: Random House; London: Hi Marketing.

>The author presents an excellent history of eating disorders, dating from the earliest days of Western civilization to the present time. She devotes one chapter to a review of recent and current methods for treatment of the disorders and one to modern dieting practices and their relationship to eating disorders.

Crisp, A. H., et al. 2014. *Anorexia Nervosa: The Wish to Change*. East Sussex and New York: Psychology Press.

>This book is designed to assist individuals with anorexia nervosa (AN) to take charge of their own efforts to deal with the condition. It contains sections on a general introduction to the condition, the 30-step program for dealing with AN, exercises that can be used in managing anorexia, and practical information for the reader's use in dealing with the condition.

Davies, Nicola, and Emma Bacon. 2017. *Eating Disorder Recovery Handbook: A Practical Guide for Long-Term Recovery*. London; Philadelphia: Jessica Kingsley Publishers.

>This book covers many detailed aspects of dealing with one's eating disorders, including understanding of one's own identity and its relationship to eating patterns, other disorders that may be associated with an eating disorder, ways of thinking about eating disorders, social aspects of eating disorders, self-help tools, and practical advice about the condition.

Donald, Helena Grace. 2017. *Learning to Love the Girl in the Mirror: A Teenage Girl's Guide to Living a Happy and Healthy Life*. Los Angeles: Torch Flame Media.

>This book is intended as a source of information as to how adolescent girls can learn to understand and accept their own body image and improve their self-esteem.

Engeln, Renee. 2017. *Beauty Sick: How the Cultural Obsession with Appearance Hurts Girls and Women*. New York: Harper-Collins Publishers.

> The author describes *beauty sickness* as "what happens when women's emotional energy gets so bound up with what they see in the mirror that it becomes harder for them to see other aspects of their lives." She devotes five sections of her book to a more comprehensive discussion of this illness, how beauty sickness affects women, how the media contributes to the development of beauty sickness, and how one can fight back against this problem.

Giordano, Simona. 2007. *Understanding Eating Disorders: Conceptual and Ethical Issues in the Treatment of Anorexia and Bulimia Nervosa*. Oxford, UK: Oxford University Press.

> The author presents a good introduction to the psychological and biological bases for the development of anorexia and bulimia. She then considers some ethical issues with regard to these conditions, such as paternalism versus respect for authority, the values of weight loss, the moral logic at the heart of eating disorders, and issues related to the law and ethics in the question of ending a person's life.

Gordon-Elliott, Janna. 2017. *Fundamentals of Diagnosing and Treating Eating Disorders: A Clinical Casebook*. Cham: Springer.

> The 16 chapters in this book are presented in the form of specific cases of individuals who "eat too little" (part one) or "eat too much" (part two). The approach to the disorders is, therefore, very personalized.

Keel, Pamela. 2017. *Eating Disorders*, 2nd ed. New York: Oxford University Press.

> This book covers a wide range of topics associated with eating disorders, including historical and cross-cultural trends, biological bases of eating disorders, pathology of conditions, prevalence, and prevention and treatment of disorders.

Lock, James, and Daniel Le Grange. 2015. *Help Your Teenager Beat an Eating Disorder*, 2nd ed. New York; London: The Guilford Press.

This book is designed for parents of young adults who may have an eating disorder, although it may well be of interest also to those teenagers. The three sections provide extensive advice on first steps in helping a teenager with an eating disorder, understanding the nature of eating disorders, and making treatment programs work.

Lock, James, and Daniel Le Grange. 2015. *Treatment Manual for Anorexia Nervosa: A Family-Based Approach*, 2nd ed. New York: Guilford Press.

This book is designed to advice therapists in their treatment of adolescents who have been diagnosed with AN, based on the authors' own clinical experience in the field. The book is organized around 20 counseling sessions that deal with all aspects of the disorder and ways in which the family can work together to help a teenager deal with his or her problem.

Monteleone, P., and F. Brambilla. 2015. "Multiple Comorbidities in People with Eating Disorders." In Sartorius, N., R. I. G. Holt, and M. Maj, eds. *Comorbidity of Mental and Physical Disorders*. Basel: Karger, 66–80.

The authors discuss the occurrence of multiple comorbidities in individuals with various types of eating disorders. They point out that conditions such as these may have profound mental and physical effects that require specific types of prevention and treatment.

Nelson, Kristen Rajczak. 2017. *Eating Disorders: When Food Is an Obsession*. New York: Lucent Press.

This book is intended for young readers, aged 12–15. It provides basic information about the most frequently mentioned eating disorders, along with sidebars describing the experiences of well-known individuals who had to deal with eating disorders.

Pope, Harrison, Katharine A. Phillips, and Roberto Olivardia. 2002. *The Adonis Complex: The Secret Crisis of Male Body Obsession.* New York; London: Simon & Schuster.

> The authors discuss various aspects of muscle dysphoria with chapters on "The Rise of the Adonis Complex," "Do You Have Adonis Complex?," "Anabolic Steroids: Dangerous Fuel for the Adonis Complex," "Beyond Muscle and Fat" (side effects of steroid use), "Boys at Risk," and "Rx for the Adonis Complex."

Robinson, Paul H., and Dasha Nicholls, eds. 2016. *Critical Care for Anorexia Nervosa.* Cham: Springer.

> The essays in this book explain the use of a program called MARSIPAN (for Management of Really Sick Patients with Anorexia Nervosa). The program was developed because of the inability of some hospital staff to deal with patients who have recurring, persistent, and/or severe cases of AN that do not respond to traditional systems of treatment.

Schmidt, Ulkike, Janet Treasure, and June Alexander. 2016. *Getting Better Bite by Bite: A Survival Kit for Sufferers of Bulimia Nervosa and Binge Eating Disorders.* Hove, East Sussex; New York: Routledge.

> This book is a very down-to-earth presentation about ways that one can deal with bulimia and binge eating. It has chapters on "Tools for the Journey," "Dieting: A Health Warning," "The Black Hole of the Insatiable Stomach," "Having Your Cake and Eating It Too," and "Learning to Feel Good about Your Body."

Schreiber, Katherine, and Heather A. Hausenblas. 2015. *The Truth about Exercise Addiction: Understanding the Dark Side of Thinspiration.* Lanham, MD: Rowman & Littlefield Publishers.

> *Exercise addiction* is defined as a person's commitment to an extreme schedule of exercise, generally for the purpose of improving one's body image. The authors explore the

nature of exercise addiction, its consequences, and its basis in "thinspiration," the strong motivation to lose weight.

Touyz, Stephen, et al., eds. 2016. *Managing Severe and Enduring Anorexia Nervosa: A Clinician's Guide*. New York: Routledge.
This book provides an excellent overview of anorexia nervosa, including chapters on "what we know" about the disorder, quality of life for individuals with the condition, managing patients who have the disorder, diagnosis and prognosis for the condition, and the use of palliative care for individuals with severe and enduring anorexia.

Treasure, Janet, Ulrike Schmidt, and Pam Macdonald. 2010. *The Clinician's Guide to Collaborative Caring in Eating Disorders: The New Maudsley Method*. London; New York: Routledge.
This important book provides a comprehensive overview of one of the most popular and most successful methods for the treatment of anorexia in adolescents.

Von Ranson, K. M. 2012. "Eating Disorder Not Otherwise Specified." In: V. S. Ramachandran, ed. *Encyclopedia of Human Behavior*, 2nd ed., vol. 2. Oxford, UK: Academic Press, 1–6.
This article provides an excellent overview of the category of eating disorders known as eating disorders not otherwise specified (EDNOS).

Wade, Tracey, ed. 2017. *Encyclopedia of Feeding and Eating Disorders*. Cham: Springer.
This set of essays discusses virtually every essential aspect of all eating disorders, incorporating new definitions and diagnostic symptoms from *DSM-V*.

Winograd, Arie M. 2016. *Face to Face with Body Dysmorphic Disorder: Psychotherapy and Clinical Insights*. New York: Taylor & Francis.
This book provides a comprehensive introduction to the topic of body dysmorphia with chapters on topics

such as how body dysmorphia begins, psychotherapy and other mechanisms for treating the condition, medication management, and intimacy and interpersonal relationships.

Young, Sera. 2012. *Craving Earth: Understanding Pica—The Urge to Eat Clay, Starch, Ice, and Chalk*. New York: Columbia University Press.

The author provides an exhaustive review of the history and features of pica, with individual chapters on topics such as who the individuals are that practice this type of eating disorder, what the medicinal value of certain types of pica-related foods may be, how pica has been a part of most major religions at one time or another, harmful effects of pica disorder, the role of pica in various slave cultures, pica as a response to food shortages, possible antitoxin effects of pica materials, and what science currently knows and doesn't know about pica.

Articles

Some journals devoted specifically to eating disorder topics:

Childhood Obesity: ISSN: 2153-2168 (Print); Online ISSN: 2153-217

Eating and Weight Disorders: 1124-4909

Eating Behaviors: ISSN: 1471-0153

European Eating Disorders Review: ISSN (Print): 1072-4133; ISSN: 1099-0968 (Online)

International Journal of Obesity: ISSN; 0307-0565

Journal of Obesity: ISSN: 2090-0708 (Print); ISSN: 2090-0716 (Online); doi10.1155/8572

Obesity: Online ISSN: 1930-739X

Obesity Reviews: Print ISSN: 1467-7881; Online ISSN: 1467-789X

Pediatric Obesity: 1747-7166 (print); 1747-7174 (Online)

Ágh, T. S., et al. 2016. "A Systematic Review of the Health-Related Quality of Life and Economic Burdens of Anorexia Nervosa, Bulimia Nervosa, and Binge Eating Disorder." *Eating and Weight Disorders.* 21(3): 353–364. https://www.ncbi.nlm.nih .gov/pmc/articles/PMC5010619/. Accessed on May 1, 2017.
    The authors conduct a review of the health-related quality of life and economic burdens of anorexia nervosa, bulimia nervosa, and binge eating disorder. They find that all conditions pose a "serious impact" on a person's quality of life and present serious economic issues for society as a whole.

Ágh, Tamás, et al. 2015. "Epidemiology, Health-Related Quality of Life and Economic Burden of Binge Eating Disorder: A Systematic Literature Review." *Eating and Weight Disorders.* 20(1): 1–12. https://www.ncbi.nlm.nih.gov/pmc/articles/PMC 4349998/. Accessed on May 1, 2017.
    This article provides a good general overview of binge eating disorder, with special attention to its effects on the lives of individuals with the condition, as well as a review of the economic impacts of the disorder in general.

Berridge, Kent C., et al. 2010. "The Tempted Brain Eats: Pleasure and Desire Circuits in Obesity and Eating Disorders." *Brain Research.* 1350: 43–64. doi:10.1016/j.brainres.2010.04.003. https://www.ncbi.nlm.nih.gov/pmc/articles/PMC2913163/. Accessed on July 13, 2017.
    The authors review the action of the human brain in the processes of "liking" and "wanting" of foods and show how these functions may be related to the development of obesity and other eating disorders.

Bert, F., et al. 2016. "Risks and Threats of Social Media Websites: Twitter and the Proana Movement." *Cyberpsychology, Behavior and Social Networking.* 19(4): 233–238. https://iris .unito.it/retrieve/handle/2318/1588562/270583/articolo_ Twitter_preprint_4aperto.pdf. Accessed on July 12, 2017.
    This study was designed to study the "presence, popularity, and content" of websites promoting anorexia. The

authors found that the web pages they studied "contain dangerous information, especially considering the young age of the users."

Bonci, Christine M., et al. 2008. "National Athletic Trainers' Association Position Statement: Preventing, Detecting, and Managing Disordered Eating in Athletes." *Journal of Athletic Training*. 43(1): 80–108.
> This position statement of the NAT is designed to assist professionals in the field of athletic training with the skills needed to diagnose and manage eating disorders among their designated population.

Bratland-Sanda, Solfrid, and Jorunn Sundgot-Borgen. 2013. "Eating Disorders in Athletes: Overview of Prevalence, Risk Factors and Recommendations for Prevention and Treatment." *European Journal of Sport Medicine*. 13(5): 499–508.
> The authors examine existing information about the occurrence of eating disorders among athletes and suggest areas for possible future research in the field.

Bray, G. A. 2004. "Obesity Is a Chronic, Relapsing Neurochemical Disease." *International Journal of Obesity*. 28(1): 34–38. http://www.nature.com/ijo/journal/v28/n1/full/0802479a.html. Accessed on May 1, 2017.
> The author provides a strong argument, based on biological and chemical events that occur in the human body, that obesity is a disease similar to other conditions now recognized as diseases, such as diabetes and cancer. Also see Heshka and Allison (2001).

Bruch, Hilde. 1962. "Perceptual and Conceptual Disturbances in Anorexia Nervosa." *Psychosomatic Medicine*. 24: 187–194.
> Bruch's paper is one of the classical documents in the history of eating disorders, one in which the full psychiatric attributes of the disorder are explored.

Casper, Regina C. 1983. "On the Emergence of Bulimia Nervosa as a Syndrome: A Historical View." *International Journal of Eating Disorders*. 2(3): 3–16.

> The author takes note that bulimia has only recently been recognized as a distinct eating disorder, especially in comparison to anorexia. She examines some of the cultural and social factors that may account for the existence and recognition of this condition.

Conceição, Eva, et al. 2013. "The Development of Eating Disorders after Bariatric Surgery." *Eating Disorders*. 21(3): 275–282.

Conceição, Eva, et al. 2013. "Eating Disorders after Bariatric Surgery: A Case Series." *International Journal of Eating Disorders*. 46(3): 274–279.

> An interesting issue that has arisen in the treatment of obesity is the emergence of eating disorders that may sometimes occur following bariatric surgery for obesity. These two articles follow the development of such events in a handful of patients to study the characteristic features of the process. The authors also conclude that the number of such cases is probably significantly underreported.

Culbert, Kristen M., Sarah E. Racine, and Kelly L. Klump. 2015. "Research Review: What We Have Learned about the Causes of Eating Disorders—A Synthesis of Sociocultural, Psychological, and Biological Research." *Journal of Child Psychology and Psychiatry*. 56(11): 1141–1164.

> The authors take on the ambitious task of summarizing research findings on the variety of factors responsible for the development of eating disorders and their interactions. They conclude that "data suggest that psychological and environmental factors interact with and influence the expression of genetic risk to cause eating pathology."

Currie, Alan, and Eric D. Morse. 2005. "Eating Disorders in Athletes: Managing the Risks." *Clinics in Sports Medicine*. 24(4): 871–883. http://users.clas.ufl.edu/msscha/whp_athletes_eatingdisorder_review.pdf. Accessed on July 12, 2017.

> The authors note that eating disorders are becoming a more common risk among athletes at all stages of proficiency. They ask a series of questions about this fact: "How likely is it that an athlete will develop an eating disorder? Who is at risk? Can eating disorders be prevented? How can athletes who have eating disorders be identified? What are the consequences of developing an eating disorder? What action can be taken to help an athlete who has an eating disorder?"

Custers, Kathleen. 2015. "The Urgent Matter of Online Pro-eating Disorder Content and Children: Clinical Practice." *European Journal of Pediatrics*. 174(4): 429–433.

> The author provides a review of the availability and appeal of so-called pro-ana websites. "Pro-ana" websites are locations that promote the concept of eating disorders such as anorexia and bulimia. The author concludes that "the dissemination of online pro-eating disorder content to different types of social networking sites is becoming an urgent issue."

Dancyger, Ida, Scott Krakower, and Victor Fornari. 2013. "Eating Disorders in Adolescents: Review of Treatment Studies That Include Psychodynamically Informed Therapy." *Child and Adolescent Psychiatric Clinics of North America*. 22(1): 97–118.

> The authors review and assess the types of psychodynamic approaches that have been and are being used in the treatment of eating disorders in adolescents.

Dickstein, L. P., et al. 2014. "Recognizing, Managing Medical Consequences of Eating Disorders in Primary Care." *Cleveland Clinic Journal of Medicine*. 81(4): 255–263.

> The authors point out that primary physicians are often the first professionals to be confronted with cases of eating

disorders. The article provides basic information on the condition and then suggests approaches that would be appropriate for a physician faced with such a condition.

Easter, Michele. 2014. "Interpreting Genetics in the Context of Eating Disorders: Evidence of Disease, Not Diversity." *Sociology of Health & Illness*. 36(6): 840–855. https://www.ncbi .nlm.nih.gov/pmc/articles/PMC4037400/. Accessed on July 7, 2017.

> The author notes that eating disorders can be understood and treated from one of two perspectives. It may be regarded as a physical or mental "disease" that can be treated, as are other types of diseases. Or it can be viewed as an inborn characteristic, the control of which may be beyond traditional types of treatments. She explores the attitudes of women who have been diagnosed (and sometimes cured) of eating disorders to see how these differing views affect their own understandings of the condition they experienced.

Foerde, Karin, et al. 2015. "Neural Mechanisms Supporting Maladaptive Food Choices in Anorexia Nervosa." *Nature Neuroscience*. 18(11): 1571–1573.

> The authors describe their research on changes in the brain that occur when people begin to reduce their food consumption. The results of this study provide additional ideas about the ways anorexia and other eating disorders can be viewed and, perhaps, treated.

Frank, Guido K. W., and Walter H. Kaye. 2012. "Current Status of Functional Imaging in Eating Disorders." *International Journal of Eating Disorders*. 45(6): 723–736.

> Functional image is a procedure in which various types of imaging technologies, such as magnetic resonance imaging, positron emission tomography, and computed tomography perfusion imaging, are used to record changes that take place in the brain during or following certain types of mental activities, such as those associated with

eating disorders. This article reviews the results of recent and current research on the technology with respect to new information gained about the etiology of eating disorders.

Gatt, Lauren, et al. 2014. "The Household Economic Burden of Eating Disorders and Adherence to Treatment in Australia." *BMC Psychiatry*. 14(1): 338–347. https://bmcpsy chiatry.biomedcentral.com/track/pdf/10.1186/s12888-014-0338-0?site=bmcpsychiatry.biomedcentral.com. Accessed on July 12, 2017.

> This article claims to be "the first to empirically and quantitatively examine the household economic burden of eating disorders from the patient perspective." The authors find that eating disorders impose a substantial economic burden on the members of a household where such conditions occur and that such burdens may actually contribute to maintenance of an eating disorder.

Ghaznavi, Jannath, and Laramie D. Taylor. 2015. "Bones, Body Parts, and Sex Appeal: An Analysis of #Thinspiration Images on Popular Social Media." *Body Image*. 14: 54–61.

> This article reports on a study of pro-eating disorder sites that promote the concept of thinness (thinspiration sites), their variability from site to site, and potential harmful effects of the concept.

Haslam, D. 2007. "Obesity: A Medical History." *Obesity Reviews*. 8(Suppl. 1): 31–36. http://onlinelibrary.wiley.com/doi/10.1111/j.1467-789X.2007.00314.x/full. Accessed on May 1, 2017.

> This article provides an excellent review of medical views about obesity from the ancient Egyptians to the present day. The author also discusses the relationship between obesity and other diseases; special issues with regard to obese women; management of the condition; and the present status of obesity research, prevention, and treatment.

Heshka, S., and D. B. Allison. 2001. "Is Obesity a Disease?" *International Journal of Obesity.* 25(10): 1401–1404. https://www.nature.com/ijo/journal/v25/n10/full/0801790a.html. Accessed on May 1, 2017.

> The authors argue that there are not adequate criteria to label obesity as a disease, although there may be nonmedical reasons for doing so. Also see Bray (2004).

Honig, Peter, and Marianne Bentovim. 2016. "Treating Children with Eating Disorders Ethical and Legal Issues." *Clinical Child Psychology and Psychiatry.* 1(2): 287–294.

> Moral and legal questions as to a person's right to consent to medical treatment may arise with children and adolescents with eating disorders. The authors review existing legal decisions on this issue and then discuss remaining legal and ethical issues with regard to this problem.

Hurst, Kim, Shelly Read, and Andrew Wallis. 2012. "Anorexia Nervosa in Adolescence and Maudsley Family-Based Treatment." *Journal of Counseling & Development.* 90(3): 339–345. http://www.theresiliencecentre.com.au/images/product/file/Anorexia-Nervosa-in-Adolescence.pdf. Accessed on July 8, 2017.

> This article provides an excellent overview of the Maudsley method of treating anorexia in adolescents. It includes a history of the procedure's development, the basic features of its implementation, and a review of efficacy studies on the approach.

Joy, Elizabeth, Andrea Kussman, and Aurelia Nattiv. 2016. "Update on Eating Disorders in Athletes: A Comprehensive Narrative Review with a Focus on Clinical Assessment and Management." *British Journal of Sports Medicine.* 50(3): 154–162. http://bjsm.bmj.com/content/50/3/154. Accessed on July 9, 2017.

> The authors summarize the most recent research on eating disorders among male and female athletes and comment

on the responsibilities of team physicians to screen for and be aware of the risk that athletes face with regard to eating disorders.

Kazdin, Alan E., et al. 2017. "Addressing Critical Gaps in the Treatment of Eating Disorders." *International Journal of Eating Disorders*. 50(3): 170–189.

The authors point out that there is a significant gap between what we know about eating disorders, based on research studies, and how that information is used in treating these conditions in the everyday world. They say that "the vast majority of individuals in need of mental health services for eating disorders and other mental health problems do not receive treatment."

Kim, Sangwon F. 2012. "Animal Models of Eating Disorders." *Neuroscience*. 211: 2–12. https://www.ncbi.nlm.nih.gov/pmc/articles/PMC3351502/. Accessed on July 7, 2017.

Given the unique features of eating disorders among humans, it might seem unrealistic to expect that such conditions can be explored in rats and other laboratory animals. To some extent, that presumption is true. Still, some researchers believe that at least some aspects of eating disorders can be studied in such settings. This article summarizes the problems involved in such studies, their potential in spite of these difficulties, and some preliminary results from animal studies of eating disorders.

Kontis, Dimitrios, and Erini Theochari. 2012. "Dopamine in Anorexia Nervosa: A Systematic Review." *Behavioural Pharmacology*. 23(5/6): 496–515.

The authors review the experimental evidence about the relationship of the neurotransmitter dopamine and the etiology of eating disorders. They report that results are ambiguous and sometimes contradictory with studies showing changes in dopamine levels increasing, decreasing, or having no relationships in individuals with eating disorders.

Loucas, Christina E., et al. 2014. "E-therapy in the Treatment and Prevention of Eating Disorders: A Systematic Review and Meta-analysis." *Behaviour Research and Therapy*. 63: 122–131.
Given the ubiquity of electronic resources available to the general public today, it should not be surprising to find that some experts in the field of eating disorders are exploring the possibility of using online programs to treat such conditions in at least some points in a treatment program and/or certain types of individuals. This article reviews the available information on the efficacy of e-therapy for eating disorders and finds it to be "uncertain."

Luiselli, James K. 2015. "Behavioral Treatment of Rumination: Research and Clinical Applications." *Journal of Applied Behavior Analysis*. 48: 707–711. doi:10.1002/jaba.221. http://www.clinicalsolutionsma.com/wp-content/uploads/2015/09/Luiselli-JABA-20152.pdf. Accessed on July 5, 2017.
The author reports on his review of recent articles on rumination, with special attention to treatment methods for the disorder.

Lupton, Deborah. 2017. "Digital Media and Body Weight, Shape, and Size: An Introduction and Review." *Fat Studies*. 6(2): 119–134.
As an introduction to a special issue on body image and the media, this study reviews the variety of ways in which overweight and obesity are represented in various parts of the media and shows that these presentations are often in stark conflict with each other.

Madowitz, Jennifer, Brittany E. Matheson, and June Llang. 2015. "The Relationship between Eating Disorders and Sexual Trauma." *Eating and Weight Disorders.* 20(3): 281–293.

> Sexual trauma is often listed as a contributing factor in the development of eating disorders. The authors review current evidence on this point and find that there is some, but limited, evidence to support the hypothesis.

Manley, Ronald S., Vicki Smye, and Suja Srikameswaran. 2001. "Addressing Complex Ethical Issues in the Treatment of Children and Adolescents with Eating Disorders: Application of a Framework for Ethical Decision-Making." *European Eating Disorders Review.* 9(3): 144–166.

> The authors point out that children and adolescents with eating disorders may develop serious, even life-threatening, health problems as a result of these practices. Clinicians may be faced with profound ethical decisions as to how to act in such cases. They recommend a framework within which such decisions can be made.

Matusek, Jill Anne, and Margaret O'Dougherty Wright. 2010. "Ethical Dilemmas in Treating Clients with Eating Disorders: A Review and Application of an Integrative Ethical Decision-Making Model." *European Eating Disorders Review.* 18(6): 434–452. http://www.marshall.edu/psych/files/2012/06/Eating-Disorders.pdf. Accessed on July 13, 2017.

> The authors explore a number of ethical issues related to the treatment of patients with eating disorders, such as "imposed treatment, enforced feeding, the duty to protect minors and adults, the determination of competence and capacity among medically comprised clients, and the effectiveness of coercive treatment for clients with eating disorder."

McElroy, Susan L., et al. 2012. "Pharmacological Management of Binge Eating Disorder: Current and Emerging

Treatment Options." *Therapeutics and Clinical Risk Management*. 8: 219–241. https://www.ncbi.nlm.nih.gov/pmc/articles/PMC3363296/. Accessed on July 6, 2017.

Research suggests that some types of pharmacotherapy may be helpful in controlling binge eating. This article reviews that research and suggests the overall conclusions as to what it suggests about the treatment of binge eating disorder.

Mishori, Ranit, and Courtney McHale. 2014. "Pica: An Age-Old Eating Disorder That's Often Missed." *The Journal of Family Practice*. 63(7): E1–E4.

This article is intended for the family physician, providing a general introduction to the diagnosis, possible outcomes, and management of the disease. An extensive bibliography provides suggestions for further reading in the field.

Mishra, Anand, Manu Anand, and Shreekantiah Umesh. 2017. "Neurobiology of Eating Disorders—An Overview." *Asian Journal of Psychiatry*. 25: 91–100.

This meta-analysis reviews the most recent evidence on the variety of brain changes that may be involved with the development of eating disorders.

Mitchell, Lachian, et al. 2017. "Muscle Dysmorphia Symptomatology and Associated Psychological Features in Bodybuilders and Non-bodybuilder Resistance Trainers: A Systematic Review and Meta-analysis." *Sports Medicine*. 47(2): 233–259. https://www.researchgate.net/publication/303711119_Muscle_Dysmorphia_Symptomatology_and_Associated_Psychological_Features_in_Bodybuilders_and_Non-Bodybuilder_Resistance_Trainers_A_Systematic_Review_and_Meta-Analysis. Accessed on July 10, 2017.

The authors studied the correlation between certain types of psychological factors and body dysmorphia in the groups of men listed in the title of the article. They found that "anxiety and social physique anxiety, depression, neuroticism, and perfectionism were positively associated with MD [muscle dysphoria], while self-concept and self-esteem were negatively associated."

Mond, Jonathan M. 2013. "Eating Disorders as 'Brain-Based Mental Illnesses': An Antidote to Stigma?" 2013. *Journal of Mental Health*. 22(1): 1–3. http://www.tandfonline.com/doi/pdf/10.3109/09638237.2012.760192?needAccess=true. Accessed on July 13, 2017.

The author notes that people with eating disorders are often stigmatized because they are seen as having weak wills or other negative attitudes about eating. He suggests that research on the biological bases of such conditions might reduce the stigmatization of those with eating disorders, and he reviews the (limited) available research on that topic.

Munn-Chernoff, Melissa A., and Jessica H. Baker. 2016. "A Primer on the Genetics of Comorbid Eating Disorders and Substance Use Disorders." *European Eating Disorders Review*. 24(2): 91–100.

This review is one of a number of studies focusing on the genetic basis for comorbidities between eating disorders and substance abuse disorders. The authors find few strong connections between the two conditions in research conducted thus far.

O'Brien, Katie M., et al. 2017. "Eating Disorders and Breast Cancer." *Cancer Epidemiology, Biomarkers & Prevention*. 26(2): 206–211.

The authors report on their study that shows that women who have or have had eating disorders have a significantly decreased likelihood of developing breast cancer.

Parry-Jones, B., and W. L. Parry-Jones. 1992. "Pica: Symptom or Eating Disorder? A Historical Assessment." *The British Journal of Psychiatry.* 160: 341–354.

> The authors observe that pica was historically considered to be a symptom of some other mental or physical disorder rather than a discrete disorder in and of itself. In this article, they trace the history of the transition from symptom to disease.

Peterson, Clair M., et al. 2016. "Genetic and Environmental Components to Self-Induced Vomiting." *International Journal of Eating Disorders.* 49(4): 421–427.

> The authors explore the etiology of a common feature of anorexia, bulimia, and binge eating disorder: self-induced vomiting. They conclude that research on the genetic basis of the practice has thus far produced no useful results, although studies on environmental influence have done so. They review some clinical implications for these findings.

Pila, Eva, et al. 2017. "A Thematic Content Analysis of #Cheatmeal Images on Social Media: Characterizing an Emerging Dietary Trend." *International Journal of Eating Disorders.* 50(6): 698–706.

> "Cheat meals" are one-time (e.g., once a week) meals at which a person splurges on food, eating as much of anything as he or she wants. The practice has been receiving increasing attention as a way of helping individuals stay on otherwise strict weight-loss diets. This study examines web portrayals of cheat meals and their possible effects on a person's weight patterns.

Ridaura, V. K., et al. 2013. "Gut Microbiota from Twins Discordant for Obesity Modulate Metabolism in Mice." *Science.* 341(6150): 1241214. doi:10.1126.

> The results of this research on mice provide a hint that intestinal bacteria may be a factor in determining weight

gain. For a layperson's overview, also see Wallis (2014) in the Internet section.

Rothenberg, Albert. 1986. "Eating Disorder as a Modern Obsessive-Compulsive Syndrome." *Psychiatry*. 49(1): 45–53. https://www.researchgate.net/publication/19698603_Eating_Disorder_as_a_Modern_Obsessive-Compulsive_Syndrome. Accessed on July 5, 2017.

> The author makes the general argument that psychiatric diagnoses are made and used to a significant extent by cultural and social factors in existence at any given time. He then goes on to show how those factors have been responsible, at least in part, to the rise in concern about eating disorders which were, for the most part, not a major concern of the medical profession prior to the mid-twentieth century.

Russell, Gerald. 1979. "Bulimia Nervosa: An Ominous Variant of Anorexia Nervosa." *Psychological Medicine*. 9(3): 429–448.

> This is one of the classic papers in the history of eating disorders, the first to suggest that bulimia is a type of eating disorder distinct from anorexia.

Steiger, Howard. 2017. "Evidence-Informed Practices in the Real-World Treatment of People with Eating Disorders." *Eating Disorders*. 25(2): 173–181. http://www.tandfonline.com/doi/full/10.1080/10640266.2016.1269558?scroll=top&needAccess=true. Accessed on July 8, 2017.

> The author notes that information about effective treatments for eating disorders is currently available, but about half of all patients who complete treatment programs can still be diagnosed with an eating disorder. He lists and discusses a number of evidence-based principles that should inform effective treatment programs for eating disorders.

Trace, Sara E., et al. 2013. "The Genetics of Eating Disorders." *Annual Review of Clinical Psychology.* 9: 589–620.

The authors provide an extensive and detailed review of the scientific literature on the genetic basis of eating disorders, with additional comments on emerging hypotheses, future directions, and clinical implications of the research.

Trent, Stacy A., et al. 2013. "ED Management of Patients with Eating Disorders." *The American Journal of Emergency Medicine.* 31(5): 859–865.

The authors point out the special problems posed to emergency department workers with the presentation of individuals having eating disorders. Signs and symptoms can often mimic those of other diseases and disorders, and a correct diagnosis of an eating disorder is essential. They suggest some practices for ED workers in helping to deal with this issue.

Van Elburg, Annemarie A., and Janet Treasure. 2013. "Advances in the Neurobiology of Eating Disorders." *Current Opinion in Psychiatry.* 26(6): 556–561.

The authors discuss the ways in which the National Institute of Mental Health's new Research Domain Criteria program can be used to provide a new mechanism for understanding the etiology of eating disorders. (See Wildes and Marcus 2015 for more details.)

Vandereycken, Walter, and Katrien Devidt. 2010. "Dropping Out from a Specialized Inpatient Treatment for Eating Disorders: The Perception of Patients and Staff." *Eating Disorders.* 18(2): 140–147.

One of the ongoing issues with treatment programs for eating disorders is the fairly high rate of dropouts from such programs. In this study, the authors explore the reasons given by staff members and by patients as to the reasons for dropouts from such programs.

Weissman, Ruth Striegel, and Francine Rosselli. 2017. "Reducing the Burden of Suffering from Eating Disorders: Unmet Treatment Needs, Cost of Illness, and the Quest for Cost-Effectiveness." *Behaviour Research and Therapy.* 88: 49–64.

This study examines three critical issues in the treatment of eating disorders: number of individuals who receive adequate treatment, cost of treatment programs, and cost-effectiveness of various programs. The authors conclude that the number of individuals who receive adequate treatment is still very low, the cost of such treatments can be prohibitively high, and major gaps exist in the cost-effectiveness of such treatment plans.

Wildes, Jennifer, E., and Marsha D. Marcus. 2015. "Application of the Research Domain Criteria (RDoC) Framework to Eating Disorders: Emerging Concepts and Research." *Current Psychiatry Reports.* 17(5): 1–10. PubMed PMID: 25773226. https://www.researchgate.net/publication/273639123_Application_of_the_Research_Domain_Criteria_RDoC_Framework_to_Eating_Disorders_Emerging_Concepts_and_Research. Accessed on July 7, 2017.

Most discussions of eating disorders, including their diagnosis and treatment, are based on a psychiatric view of the conditions, as outlined specifically in the *Diagnostic and Statistical Manual of Mental Disorders.* Over the past decade, the National Institute of Mental Health has proposed a different model for studying mental disorders, including eating disorders. The Research Domain Criteria assumes that mental disorders have discrete and identifiable biological etiologies centered in molecular, genetic, neurobiological, cellular, or other features. This article discusses the ways in which this new approach to the study of mental disorders has been and can be applied to the study of eating disorders.

Woolley, Dawn. 2017. "Aberrant Consumers: Selfies and Fat Admiration Websites." *Fat Studies*. 6(2): 206–222.

> The author takes note of the conflict between healthy (usually slender) bodies and motivation for instant gratification, both provided by the Internet and other media sources. The author argues that the inability of some individuals to balance these two forces accounts for the rise in abnormally thin or fat bodies in today's society.

Zimmerman, Jacqueline, and Martin Fisher. 2017. "Avoidant/ Restrictive Food Intake Disorder (ARFID)." *Current Problems in Pediatric and Adolescent Health Care*. 47(4): 95–103.

> The authors introduce and explain this new category of eating disorders. They explain how the classification differs from the previous "Feeding Disorder of Infancy or Early Childhood," as defined in *DSM-IV*. They also summarize what is currently known about the condition and, in much greater quantity, what still needs to be researched.

Reports

Academy for Eating Disorders. 2012. "Eating Disorders: Critical Points for Early Recognition and Medical Risk Management in the Care of Individuals with Eating Disorders," 2nd ed. Deerfield, IL: Academy for Eating Disorders. https:// higherlogicdownload.s3.amazonaws.com/AEDWEB/05 656ea0-59c9-4dd4-b832-07a3fea58f4c/UploadedImages/ AED_Medical_Care_Guidelines_English_04_03_18_a.pdf. Accessed on November 28, 2018.

> This report is designed as "a resource to promote recognition and prevention of medical morbidity and mortality associated with eating disorders." Discrete sections focus on topics such as key guidelines, important facts about eating disorders, presenting signs and symptoms, early recognition, a comprehensive assessment, refeeding syndrome, goals of treatment, timely interventions, and ongoing management.

Berkman, Nancy D., et al. 2015. "Management and Outcomes of Binge-Eating Disorder." Rockville, MD: Agency for Healthcare Research and Quality. U.S. Department of Health and Human Services. *Comparative Effectiveness Review*, no. 160; AHRQ publication, no. 15(16)-EHC030-EF. https://www.ncbi.nlm.nih.gov/pubmedhealth/PMH0084317/pdf/PubMed Health_PMH0084317.pdf. Accessed on May 1, 2017.

>   This document reviews information about the treatment of binge eating disorder and related conditions collected from a detailed examination of literature on the topic. The report is part of the AHRQ program on evidence-based treatment for a variety of diseases and other conditions.

"The Costs of Eating Disorders: Social, Health and Economic Impacts." 2015. PWC (Pricewaterhouse Cooper) for BEAT (Beating Eating Disorders). https://www.beateatingdisorders.org.uk/uploads/documents/2017/10/the-costs-of-eating-disorders-final-original.pdf. Accessed on November 28, 2018.

>   This study in the United Kingdom assessed the financial costs to families in which at least one individual had been diagnosed with an eating disorder. The extensive data obtained led researchers to the conclusion that although "you can't put a price against a life," what the report shows is that there is "a crucial window of opportunity that can make all the difference between an early recovery and the devastating effects of a long-term illness."

Darvell, Marcia, and British Medical Association. 2000. *Eating Disorders, Body Image & the Media*. London: British Medical Association, Board of Science and Education.

>   This report is an excellent, if now somewhat dated, overview of the nature of eating disorders, their etiology, the role played by the media in their development, and some recommendations for reducing adverse effects of the media on eating habits.

Devlin, Eamann. 2016. "Report on Eating Disorders—Children and Young People." Health Overview and Scrutiny Committee. Barnet London Borough. https://barnet.moderngov. co.uk/documents/s31721/Eating%20Disorders%20-%20Chil dren%20and%20Young%20People.pdf. Accessed on July 10, 2017.

> This document is of particular interest because it focuses on eating disorder issues for a very specific region, the borough of Barnet, in London. It provides information on the status of the disorder within the boundaries of the borough and outlines the steps the local government can take to deal with the problem.

Division of Adolescent and School Health, National Center for Chronic Disease Prevention and Health Promotion. 2011. "School Health Guidelines to Promote Healthy Eating and Physical Activity." *Morbidity and Mortality Weekly Report.* 60(5): whole. https://www.cdc.gov/mmwr/pdf/rr/rr6005.pdf. Accessed on July 10, 2017.

> This report summarizes practices in all 50 states and the District of Columbia on policies and practices developed by school districts to encourage the types of eating and exercise habits that can contribute to a reduced rate of obesity in children and adolescents in the United States. The report includes nearly 700 references on this topic.

"Eating Disorder Statistics." 2017. ANAD. http://www.anad .org/get-information/about-eating-disorders/eating-disorders-statistics/. Accessed on July 9, 2017.

> Although valid and reliable statistics on eating disorders are difficult to obtain, this report does an excellent job of summarizing some of the best data that are available about the prevalence and incidence of eating disorders.

"Eating Disorders among Girls and Women in Canada." 2014. Report of the Standing Committee on the Status of

Women. https://nedic.ca/sites/default/files//Status%20of%20 Women%20Report%20Eating%20Disorders.pdf. Accessed on July 10, 2017.

> This report is the fourth in a series of such documents on the status of eating disorders in Canada. The report focuses, in particular, on the factors that lead to eating disorders and the obstacles in obtaining treatment for the disorders. For an interesting commentary on this report, also see "Parliamentary Committee Report on Eating Disorders Disappoints Advocates" at http://globalnews. ca/news/1696499/parliamentary-committee-report-on-eating-disorders-disappoints-advocate/.

Hudson, James I., et al. 2007. "The Prevalence and Correlates of Eating Disorders in the National Comorbidity Survey Replication." *Biological Psychiatry.* 61(3): 348–358. doi:10.1016/j. biopsych.2006.03.040. https://www.ncbi.nlm.nih.gov/pmc/ articles/PMC1892232/?TB_iframe=true&width=921.6&hei ght=921.6. Accessed on July 9, 2017.

> Few data are available on the comorbidities associated with eating disorders. This article summarizes the result of a study on this question based on the National Comorbidity Survey Replication. The authors conclude that "eating disorders, although relatively uncommon, represent a public health concern because they are frequently associated with other psychopathology and role impairment, and are frequently under-treated."

Joint Commission on Health Care Healthy Living/Health Services Subcommittee. 2011. "Study of Eating Disorders in the Commonwealth." Summary of report is available at http://ser vices.dlas.virginia.gov/User_db/frmView.aspx?ViewId=1993. Accessed on July 10, 2017.

> In 2010, the state senate of Virginia directed the Joint Commission on Health Care to conduct a study of eating disorder issues in the state. This PowerPoint presentation

summarizes the detailed findings about the status of eating disorders in the state along with four policy options for dealing with the problem. An excellent overview of the condition for one specific state in the Union.

May, Ashleigh L., et al. "Obesity—United States, 1999–2010." 2013. *Morbidity and Mortality Weekly*. 62(3): 120–128. https://www.cdc.gov/mmwr/preview/mmwrhtml/su6203a20.htm?s_cid=su6203a20_e. Accessed on July 10, 2017.

This report provides extensive statistical data on the prevalence, incidence, and nature of obesity among the general population and special groups within the United States between 1999 and 2010. The report concludes that "although the rate of obesity has plateaued in recent years for some groups, the overall prevalence of the condition remains high for all U.S. residents, and disparities persist in the prevalence of obesity."

"Nutrition, Physical Activity, and Obesity." 2015. Centers for Disease Control and Prevention. https://www.cdc.gov/psr/2013/npao/index.html. Accessed on July 9, 2017.

This website is a section from the 2013 edition of the CDC's "Prevention Status Reports" dealing with eating disorders. It included statistics, data, and information on policies and practices in secondary schools, state nutrition standards for foods and beverages, inclusion of nutrition and physical activity in licensed childcare facilities, required physical education time in the states, and average birth facility score for breastfeeding support.

"Paying the Price: The Economic and Social Impact of Eating Disorders in Australia." 2012. The Butterfly Foundation. https://www.deloitteaccesseconomics.com.au/uploads/File/Butterfly_Report_Paying%20the%20Price_online.pdf. Accessed on July 12, 2017.

This exhaustive report covers the economic and social costs to individuals, families, and the general society of eating disorders in Australia. It contains detailed information on a host of topics, such as health costs, productivity costs, carer costs, and other financial costs.

Rosen, David S., and the Committee on Adolescence. 2010. "Clinical Report—Identification and Management of Eating Disorders in Children and Adolescents." *Pediatrics*. 126(6): 1240–1253. http://pediatrics.aappublications.org/content/pe diatrics/early/2010/11/29/peds.2010-2821.full.pdf. Accessed on July 10, 2017.
 This report discusses the diagnostic criteria for various types of eating disorders along with the range of treatment options that are available in the field.

Samnalieva, Mihail, et al. 2015. "The Economic Burden of Eating Disorders and Related Mental Health Comorbidities: An Exploratory Analysis Using the U.S. Medical Expenditures Panel Survey." *Preventive Medicine Reports*. 2: 32–34. http://ac.els-cdn.com/S2211335514000230/1-s2.0-S22113 35514000230-main.pdf?_tid=c0527184-64c7-11e7-83ba-00000aacb35f&acdnat=1499619654_cb7f436f0a8436ed 99836b5817d7769c. Accessed on July 9, 2017.
 Relatively little is known about the economic burden (economic consequences) of eating disorders and their comorbidities. This report provides some important basic data on the question. Individuals with eating disorders have significantly higher health expenses per year than do those without eating disorders. But they have no other statistically different economic consequences of the condition than do those without eating disorders.

Zhao, Yafu, and William Encinosa. 2009. "Hospitalizations for Eating Disorders from 1999 to 2006." Statistical Brief #70. Agency for Healthcare Research and Quality.

https://www.hcup-us.ahrq.gov/reports/statbriefs/sb70.pdf. Accessed on July 9, 2017.

> Although now somewhat dated, this report provides excellent baseline data on rates and categories of hospitalizations for patients with eating disorders in the United States.

Internet

Absah, I., et al. 2017. "Rumination Syndrome: Pathophysiology, Diagnosis, and Treatment." *Neurogastroenterology & Motility*. 29(4). e12954. doi:10.1111/nmo.12954. http://onlinelibrary.wiley.com/doi/10.1111/nmo.12954/full. Accessed on July 5, 2017.

> Although somewhat technical, this article provides an excellent general overview of psychiatry's current understanding of the causes, effects, and treatment of ruminant disorder, along with suggestions for its differential diagnosis.

Adaes, Sara. 2016. "The Neurobiology of Anorexia Nervosa." BrainBlogger. http://brainblogger.com/2016/01/21/the-neurobiology-of-anorexia-nervosa/. Accessed on July 8, 2017.

> This article provides a good general introduction to brain changes that may be responsible for the development of eating disorders. A good list of references is included.

Aguglia, Regis. 2017. "A Focus on Body Image & Eating Disorders in Boys & Men for #menshealthmonth." The Center for Eating Disorders at Sheppard Pratt. https://eatingdisorder.org/blog/2017/06/a-focus-on-body-image-eating-disorders-in-boys-men-for-menshealthmonth/. Accessed on July 11, 2017.

> The writer reviews some of the current research on the connections between body image and eating disorders among males, along with some suggestions for ways of dealing with that problem.

Angyal, Chloe. 2013. "The 'Thinspiration' behind an Impossible Ideal of Beauty." *Nation*. https://www.thenation.com/article/thinspiration-behind-impossible-ideal-beauty/. Accessed on July 12, 2017.

> The author comments on the phenomenon of "thinspiration," a movement that encourages poor eating habits, supposedly as a way of improving one's body image and sexual attraction.

Arnold, Carrie. 2016. "The Challenge of Treating Anorexia in Adults." *Atlantic*. https://www.theatlantic.com/health/archive/2016/03/treating-anorexia-in-adults/475845/. Accessed on May 2, 2017.

> This article provides a brief review of the history of anorexia and then discusses changes in the way the disorders have been viewed by specialists in the field and the general public. It also discusses some of the most recent methods of treatment used for the disorder.

Bernstein, Bettina. 2017. "Binge-Eating Disorder." Medscape. http://emedicine.medscape.com/article/2221362-overview#showall. Accessed on May 1, 2017.

> This article provides an excellent general overview of binge eating that includes a discussion of its anatomical and pathophysiological features along with its etiology, epidemiology, treatment, prognosis, and patient education about the condition.

Birch, Jenna. 2017. Self. http://www.self.com/story/10-subtle-signs-someone-you-love-might-have-an-eating-disorder. Accessed on May 7, 2017.

> This website provides an insight into some subtle signs that a friend or family member may have an eating disorder. Its special feature is that it lists some items that are not generally mentioned in other web pages on this topic.

Brown, Tiffany A., and Pamela K. Keel. 2012. "Current and Emerging Directions in the Treatment of Eating Disorders."

Substance Abuse: Research and Treatment. 6: 33–61. doi:10.4137/
SART.S7864. https://www.ncbi.nlm.nih.gov/pmc/articles/PMC
3411516/. Accessed on July 8, 2017.
> This lengthy article summarizes some of the most recent
> information available on the options available for the
> treatment of various eating disorders and the relative ef-
> fectiveness of each option for each eating disorder.

Collins, Sam P. K. 2015. "Missouri Becomes First State to
Expand Insurance Coverage for Eating Disorders." Think
Progress. https://thinkprogress.org/missouri-becomes-the-first-
state-to-expand-insurance-coverage-for-eating-disorders-
1ddc4e48949c. Accessed on July 13, 2017.
> In 2015, Missouri became the first state to require health
> insurance providers doing business in the state to cover
> the cost of certain expenses related to the treatment of eat-
> ing disorders. This article provides a review of the process
> by which that bill was passed.

Crow, Scott. 2014. "The Economics of Eating Disorder Treatment." *Current Psychiatry Reports.* 16: 454. https://link.springer
.com/article/10.1007%2Fs11920-014-0454-z. Accessed on
July 14, 2017.
> This short article reviews recent studies done on the eco-
> nomic costs of eating disorders. Those studies have fo-
> cused largely on the national costs of eating disorders,
> third-party payer costs for treatment, societal costs, and
> cost-effectiveness analysis of specific treatments.

"The Dollars and Cents of Eating Disorders." 2014. Science of
Eating Disorders. http://www.scienceofeds.org/2014/06/26/
the-dollars-and-cents-of-eating-disorders/. Accessed on July 14,
2017.
> The author provides an excellent review of recent studies
> on the economics of eating disorders. The article is help-
> ful because of its links to some of the most important of
> those studies on specific aspects of the general question as

to how much treatments for eating disorders cost (both to caregivers and to the society at large).

"Dopamine and Anorexia Nervosa: Tackling the Myths." 2013. Science of Eating Disorders. http://www.scienceofeds .org/2013/01/05/dopamine-and-anorexia-nervosa-tackling-the-myths-part-1-intro/. Accessed on July 12, 2017.

This article is the first of four in which the author explains the theory that dopamine may be involved in the onset of eating disorders and then reviews existing evidence in support of (or against) this theory. The last article in the series deals with the use of antipsychotics in the treatment of eating disorders.

Ekern, Jacquelyn. 2017. "Binge Eating Disorder: Causes, Symptoms, Signs & Treatment Help." Eating Disorder Hope. https://www.eatingdisorderhope.com/information/binge-eat ing-disorder#Signs-amp-Symptoms-of-Binge-Eating-Disor der. Accessed on May 7, 2017.

This web article is an especially good source of information about binge eating, not only because of the article itself but also because of the extensive list of other resources on the subject at the conclusion of the article.

Fassino, Secondo, and Giovanni Abbate-Data. 2013. "Resistance to Treatment in Eating Disorders: A Critical Challenge." *BMC Psychiatry*. 13: 282. doi:10.1186/1471-244X-13-282. https:// bmcpsychiatry.biomedcentral.com/articles/10.1186/1471-244X-13-282. Accessed on July 8, 2017.

This essay provides an introduction to a special issue of *BMC Psychiatry* on the phenomenon of resistance to treatment for eating disorders, with an overview of the main issues involved with this problem and the approaches suggested by the papers in the issue.

Gluck, Samantha. 2017. "What Is Muscle Dysphoria, Bigorexia, or Reverse Anorexia?" Healthy Place. https://www.healthy

place.com/ocd-related-disorders/body-dysmorphic-disorder/
what-is-muscle-dysmorphia-bigorexia-reverse-anorexia/. Accessed
on July 10, 2017.

> This article provides a good general introduction to the
> topic of muscle dysphoria or, as it is sometimes also called,
> bigorexia or reverse anorexia.

Halmi, Katherine A. 2013. "Perplexities of Treatment Resistance in Eating Disorders." *BMC Psychiatry*. 13: 292. doi:
10.1186/1471-244X-13-292. https://bmcpsychiatry.biomed
central.com/articles/10.1186/1471-244X-13-292. Accessed on
July 8, 2017.

> The author examines the question as to why it is that a
> significant number of individuals with an eating disorder
> tend to deny the nature of their condition and decline to
> participate in treatment programs. A good review of the
> relevant literature is included.

Horan, Michelle. 2010. "The Anti-ana." Artifacts. University
of Missouri. https://artifactsjournal.missouri.edu/2010/01/the-
anti-ana/. Accessed on July 12, 2017.

> In addition to providing a good general introduction to
> the topic of pro-ana and pro-mia websites, the author dis-
> cusses the question as to whether and/or to what extent
> such websites are protected by First Amendment rights
> of free speech. She concludes that "eating disorders are
> not choices; they are psychological diseases that are ge-
> netically linked and worsened by stimulus. These sites are
> extremely triggering, and for those who are suffering the
> alluring collection of photos, posts, and 'understanding'
> peers can be too hard to resist."

Hudgens, Jessica. 2015. "What I Wish Insurance Companies
Knew about Eating Disorders." Healthy Place. https://www

.healthyplace.com/blogs/survivinged/2015/07/what-i-wish-insurance-companies-understood-about-eating-disorders/. Accessed on July 13, 2017.

A woman with an eating disorder explains the problems associated with having health insurance companies pay for eating disorder treatments and the changes they could make to alleviate that problem.

"Is Eating Disorder Prevention Possible?" 2014. Science of Eating Disorders. http://www.scienceofeds.org/2014/01/15/is-eating-disorder-prevention-possible/. Accessed on July 12, 2017.

The writer presents a good overview of the literature on prevention programs for eating disorders, assesses the efficacy of such programs, and recommends some future directions for dealing with the issue.

Karimipour, Nicki. 2015. "Are Social Media Sites the New Pro-Eating Disorder Communities?" AdiosBarbie. http://www.adiosbarbie.com/2015/09/are-social-media-sites-the-new-pro-eating-disorder-communities/. Accessed on July 8, 2017.

The author discusses the role of social media in affecting views about eating disorders, with special attention to the question as to how and to what extent they may encourage young women and men to develop such practices.

Kulkarni, Shefali S. 2012. "Patients Often Find Getting Coverage for Eating Disorders Is Tough." Kaiser Health News. http://khn.org/news/binge-eating-disorder-insurance-coverage/. Accessed on July 13, 2017.

The author reviews the level of care needed by individuals being treated for eating disorders and the reasons that typical health insurance plans are unlikely to cover all or a major share of the financial costs involved.

"Legislation." 2016. National Eating Disorders Association. https://www.nationaleatingdisorders.org/tags/legislation. Accessed on July 13, 2017.

> This website provides an overview of (admittedly limited) recent and pending legislation at the federal and state levels as of mid-2017.

Maher, Hailey. 2016. "This Is Why Social Media Websites Are Having Trouble Combating Eating Disorders." Spoon University. https://spoonuniversity.com/lifestyle/this-is-why-social-media-websites-are-having-trouble-combating-eating-disorders. Accessed on July 11, 2017.

> The growth of pro-anorexia and pro-bulimia websites over the past decade has been a matter of concern to clinicians attempting to prevent or treat the conditions. They have been able to gain the cooperation of the owners of social websites in their campaign to reduce the impact of such websites. This article explains those efforts have had less success than one might hope.

Mariani, Mike. 2016. "How Pro-anorexia Website Exacerbate the Eating Disorder Epidemic." *Newsweek*. http://www.newsweek.com/2016/07/01/pro-ana-websites-anorexia-nervosa-473433.html. Accessed on May 2, 2017.

> The author comments on the presence of websites that promote behaviors associated with eating disorders and how those websites contribute to young adults' interest in and use of weight-loss practices.

Mascarelli, Amanda Leigh. 2014. "Eating Disorders: The Brain's Foul Trickery." Science News for Students. https://www.sciencenewsforstudents.org/article/eating-disorders-brain%E2%80%99s-foul-trickery/. Accessed on July 13, 2017.

> This article discusses the brain's involvement in the development of eating disorders at a level that is easily understandable to the average person.

"Maudsley Parents." 2017. http://www.maudsleyparents.org/whatismaudsley.html. Accessed on July 8, 2017.

The Maudsley approach, also known as family-based therapy, is one of the best-known and most widely used methods for treating adolescents with anorexia. The procedure was developed at Maudsley Hospital in London, from which it gets its name. This website provides a general overview of the philosophy behind the approach and the elements involved in its practice.

Mousa, Hayat M., Mary Montgomery, and Anthony Alioto. 2014. "Adolescent Rumination Syndrome." *Current Gastroenterology Reports.* 16: 398. doi:10.1007/s11894-014-0398-9.https://link.springer.com/article/10.1007/s11894-014-0398-9. Accessed on July 5, 2017.

The authors point out that rumination disorder often goes unrecognized by a primary physician. They then note that, while the disorder is not life threatening, it can have significant medical consequences. The article contains suggestions for diagnosis and treatment.

"Neurotransmitters." 2016. National Eating Disorders Association. https://www.nationaleatingdisorders.org/toolkit/parent-toolkit/neurotransmitters/ Accessed on July 13, 2017.

This short article provides an excellent and understandable overview of current information on the relationship of neurotransmitters in the etiology of eating disorders. A good bibliography is included.

Nordqvist, Christian. 2015. "Anorexia Nervosa: Causes, Symptoms and Treatments." Medical News Today. http://www.medicalnewstoday.com/articles/267432.php. Accessed on May 2, 2017.

This article provides a good general introduction to the subject of AN, including sections on its causes, symptoms, diagnosis, treatment, and complications. The article also contains a number of links to other Medical News Today articles on more specific aspects of the issue.

O'Toole, Julie. 2016. "Avoidant Restrictive Food Intake Disorder (ARFID)." Kartini Clinic. https://www.kartiniclinic.com/blog/post/avoidant-restrictive-food-intake-disorder-arfid/. Accessed on July 14, 2017.

This article provides a very personalized discussion of the nature of ARFID and some aspects of its treatment.

"Overweight and Obesity." 2017. Centers for Disease Control and Prevention. https://www.cdc.gov/obesity/. Accessed on May 3, 2017.

This website provides an excellent general introduction to the topic of overweight and obesity, with separate sections on data and statistics, childhood overweight and obesity, adult overweight and obesity, healthy food environments, and strategies to prevent obesity.

"Overweight and Obesity." 2017. National Heart, Lung, and Blood Institute. https://www.nhlbi.nih.gov/health/health-topics/topics/obe. Accessed on May 3, 2017.

This outstanding website contains individual sections on causes; risk factors; screening and prevention; signs, symptoms, and complications; diagnosis; treatment; living with; and research. It is an excellent place to begin one's study of overweight and obesity.

Pekar, Tetyana. 2016. "Why I No Longer Support Studying the Genetics of Eating Disorders." Parts 1 and 2. Science of Eating Disorders. http://www.scienceofeds.org/2016/09/09/why-i-no-longer-support-studying-the-genetics-of-eating-disorders-part-I/ and http://www.scienceofeds.org/2016/09/14/why-i-no-longer-support-genetics-research-into-eating-disorders-part-ii-illness-and-recovery-in-a-neoliberal-society. Accessed on July 7, 2017.

The author argues that spending money on research designed to identify the genetic origins of eating disorders may be misguided because it detracts attention from the substantial information we already have about ways of preventing and treating such conditions.

"Reflections on the Weight Stigma Conference 2016." 2016. Science of Eating Disorders. http://www.scienceofeds .org/2016/05/02/reflections-on-the-weight-stigma-confer ence-2016/. Accessed on July 11, 2017.
     This interesting article discusses the relationship between body dysmorphia/obesity and eating disorders with a re-view of speeches and discussions about the topic at the fourth annual Weight Stigma Conference.

Rojas, Marcela. 2014. "Social Media Helps Fuel Some Eat-ing Disorders." *USA Today*. https://www.usatoday.com/story/ news/nation/2014/06/01/social-media-helps-fuel-eating-dis orders/9817513/. Accessed on July 11, 2017.
     The author explains how pro-anorexia and pro-bulimia proponents use social media to advance their cause of en-couraging eating disorders, especially among adolescents. She also describes some ways in which therapists are at-tempting to fight back against the movement, also using social media as one of their tools.

Saber, Alan. 2016. "Obesity Surgery (Bariatric Surgery)." emedicine.com. http://www.emedicinehealth.com/surgery_in_ the_treatment_of_obesity/article_em.htm. Accessed on July 6, 2017.
     This website provides an excellent and comprehensive re-view of the procedure of bariatric surgery, conditions in which such a procedure might be indicated, technology of the procedure, benefits and risks, and postoperative care and side effects of the procedure.

Saetta, Ally. n.d. "Muscle Dysmorphia: Under-Researched and Potentially Over-Diagnosed." Barts and The London, School of Medicine and Dentistry, Queen Mary University of

London. https://www.rcpsych.ac.uk/pdf/Ally%20Saetta%20-%20Muscle%20Dysmorphia.pdf. Accessed on July 10, 2017.

This paper is one of the most thoroughly researched discussion of the nature of muscle dysphoria, its possible etiologies and characteristics, and reasons that it actually may be "overdiagnosed."

Sagan, Aleksandra. 2015. "Pro-anorexia, Bulimia Communities Thriving Online." CBC News. http://www.cbc.ca/news/health/pro-anorexia-bulimia-communities-thriving-online-1.2956149. Accessed on July 11, 2017.

This website provides examples from real life of pro-anorexia and pro-bulimia websites with reviews of some of the most popular of those websites. Of particular interest are the 275 comments made in response to this article.

"Science of Eating Disorders." 2017. http://www.scienceofeds.org/. Accessed on July 11, 2017.

This website is a gold mine of information and opinion about essentially every aspect of eating disorder research. The specific blogs are classified according to their main topic: causes and contributors, cross-cultural, genetics, medicine and physiology, neuroscience, perspectives, prevention, proana, psychiatry, psychology, public understanding, sexuality and gender, and treatment and recovery. It is a resource to be recommended to anyone researching any one of these aspects of eating disorders.

"17 Scarey Body Dysmorphic Disorder Statistics." 2014. HealthResearchFunding.org. http://healthresearchfunding.org/scarey-body-dysmorphic-disorder-statistics/. Accessed on July 11, 2017.

This article does not really have 17 "scarey statistics" about body dysmorphia, although it does have some interesting historical facts and information about the condition worth reading about. It also contains a good general discussion of the condition.

Social Media Collective. 2012. "Is Blocking Pro-ED Content the Right Way to Solve Eating Disorders?" Social Media Collective Research Blog. https://socialmediacollective.org/2012/02/24/is-blocking-pro-ed-content-the-right-way-to-solve-eating-disorders/. Accessed on July 11, 2017.
     Administrators of social media sites have become increasingly concerned about their use to promote the desirability of eating disorders. Some have attempted to block such websites, thus far without much success. This blog posting describes the efforts of Tumblr along these lines and explains why its success thus far has been less than encouraging.

Steiner, Andy. 2017. "Kitty Westin: Anna Westin Act's Passage Brings Relief, Renewed Determination." MinnPost. https://www.minnpost.com/mental-health-addiction/2017/01/kitty-westin-anna-westin-act-s-passage-brings-relief-renewed-de termi. Accessed on July 13, 2017.
     This article reports on an interview with Kitty Westin, the mother of Anna Westin, a woman who died of an eating disorder and for whom the first U.S. federal law was passed in 2016. Westin relates the circumstances under which the act was introduced and eventually passed, as well as the benefits it is likely to bring for individuals with eating disorders.

Steinglass, Joanna E., and B. Timothy Walsh. 2016. "Neurobiological Model of the Persistence of Anorexia Nervosa." *Journal of Eating Disorders*. 4: 19. doi:10.1186/s40337-016-0106-2. https://www.ncbi.nlm.nih.gov/pmc/articles/PMC4870737/. Accessed on November 28, 2018.
     The authors review the findings of latest research on changes that take place in the brain when one begins a

program of restrictive eating and how those changes tend to cause the perpetuation of the eating pattern.

"Totally in Control." 2017. Social Issues Research Center. http://www.sirc.org/articles/totally_in_control2.shtml. Accessed on July 12, 2017.

This article provides an excellent introduction to the topic of pro-anorexia and pro-bulimia websites. It discusses such issues as what the terms *pro-ana* and *pro-mia* mean specifically, what the content of these websites is, to what extent (if any) the sites promote self-harm, and the extent to which such sites are being monitored and/or censored.

Wallis, Claudia. 2014. "How Gut Bacteria Help Make Us Fat and Thin." *Scientific American.* https://www.scientificamerican .com/article/how-gut-bacteria-help-make-us-fat-and-thin/. Accessed on May 3, 2017.

This article reviews recent research that suggests that the presence or absence and/or activity of intestinal bacteria may affect a person's tendency to gain weight. (Also see Ridaura et al. 2013, in Articles.)

Warmflash, David. 2015. "You Are What You Don't Eat: Genetics of Anorexia and Bulimia." Genetics Literacy Project. https://www.geneticliteracyproject.org/2015/02/23/you-are-what-you-don't-eat-genetics-of-anorexia-and-bulimia-ner vosa/. Accessed on May 2, 2017.

This web page provides a good general introduction to the subject of genetic factors in the development of eating disorders.

Warren, Jane, and Jeffrey McGee. 2013. "Ethical Issues in Eating Disorders Treatment: Four Illustrative Scenarios." American Counseling Association VISTAS Online. http://www.coun seling.org/docs/default-source/vistas/ethical-issues-in-eating-

disorders-treatment-four-illustrative-scenarios.pdf?sfvrsn=e8a
101a9_10. Accessed on July 13, 2017.

> This article reviews some of the ethical dilemmas faced by
> counselors in their work with individuals with eating dis-
> orders. They discuss ways in which established JCA Code
> of Ethics can help guide a professional's attempts to deal
> with these issues.

Weir, Kirsten. 2016. "New Insights on Eating Disorders." American Psychological Association. http://www.apa.org/monitor/
2016/04/eating-disorders.aspx. Accessed on May 2, 2017.

> This article brings together much of the current research
> on anorexia, which shows that the condition has very spe-
> cific and identifiable neurobiological characteristics.

"What Is Body Image?" 2017. National Eating Disorders Collaboration. http://www.nedc.com.au/body-image. Accessed on
July 11, 2017.

> This website provides a good general introduction to the
> ways in which body image impacts a person's eating habits
> and some ways in which one can modify those habits to
> lead a healthier life.

"What Is Eating Disorder Not Otherwise Specified (EDNOS)?"
2014. National Eating Disorders Collaboration. http://www
.nedc.com.au/ednos. Accessed on July 5, 2017.

> This web page provides an excellent overview of EDNOS,
> along with warning signs, possible physical and mental
> effects, and treatment options.

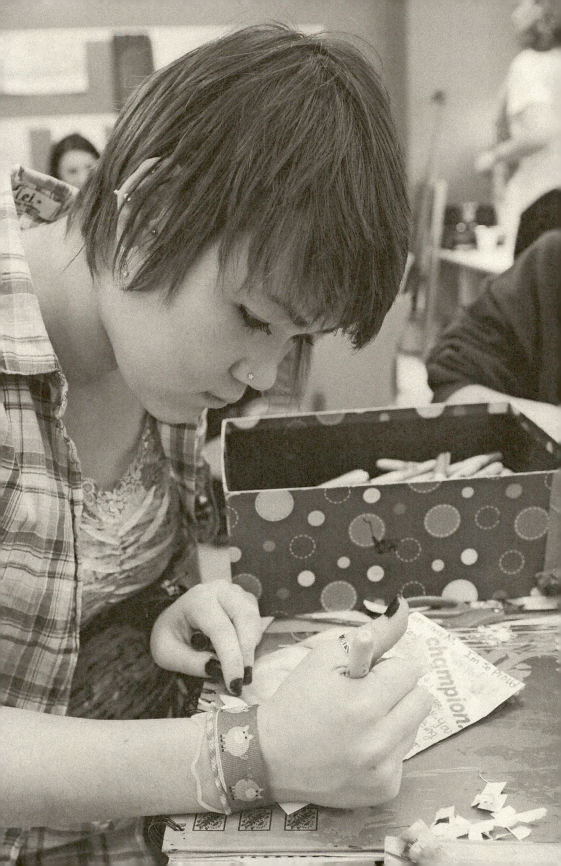

Introduction

The story of eating disorders among humans has a long and intriguing history that dates to the late Paleolithic era. Examples of anorexia nervosa, bulimia nervosa, obesity, and other eating disorders can be found at almost any point in history and almost anywhere in the world. The following chronology lists some of the most important and interesting of the events that make up that history.

ca. 1440–450 BCE   A number of references to fasting during this biblical period are available, often as a mechanism by which a person could have visions about some important concept or event. For example, Moses fasted for 40 days before receiving the Ten Commandments, Jesus fasted for 40 days in the wilderness, and Elijah fasted for 40 days while walking to Mount Horeb.

Sixth century BCE   Seer Vardhamana Mahavira, founder of the Jain religion, commits suicide by starving himself to death. The act was one of the ways in which a person could separate

An eating disorder patient works on her art therapy book during a session at the Ponzio Creative Arts Therapy Program in Denver, Colorado. The Ponzio Creative Arts Therapy Program offers art, dance/movement, music, and yoga therapies that help children identify, explore, and transform emotional and psychological difficulties. (Andy Cross/The Denver Post via Getty Images) one's earthly body from his or her eternal soul. Members of the sect continue the practice today. (*See also* **2015**.)

ca. 430 BCE   The Greek historian, Herodotus, writes in book two, chapter 77, of his *Histories*, that the Egyptians have a practice of purging on three consecutive days each month. The practice is based on their belief that food is the basic cause of all human disease.

ca. 300 BCE   Self-starvation is employed by Greek men for a variety of reasons. For example, it is said that the philosophers Cleanthes, Democritus, and Dionysius all committed suicide by self-starvation. The practice was also sometimes used because of illegal or immoral activities. Such was the case with Athenaeus, who starved himself to death after having been convicted of embezzlement. Self-starvation was reputedly a common practice among early Greek hermits, who saw it as a way of escaping from the distracting events of everyday life.

ca. 100–400 CE   Self-starvation becomes a common practice among early Christian monks, who believe that pleasures of the flesh, such as eating and drinking, reduce the likelihood of one's salvation after death. A prominent example is Saint Simeon Stylites, who isolated himself for 37 years on top of a tall pillar near the modern-day city of Aleppo. He is said to have survived on milk and bread provided to him by citizens who passed the nourishment to him by rope.

383 CE   A Roman woman of the aristocracy, aged 20 and a follower of Saint Jerome (ca. 347–420), dies as a result of self-starvation, which he preached as essential to purity and salvation. (Jerome then fled to Bethlehem, where he lived for the rest of his life in a cave translating the Bible from Hebrew and Greek into Latin.) The death of the woman is sometimes cited as the first fatality that can be traced to anorexia nervosa, although that condition had not yet been formally recognized and named.

ca. 500–1000   During the period of the so-called Dark Ages, there are relatively few reports of self-starvation among ordinary people. A number of (almost all) female saints of the Roman Catholic Church from that period, however, are said to have died in the pursuit of holiness and purity because of, or at least partly because of, self-starvation. They included Saints Catherine of Sienna, Domenica dal Paradiso, Juliana, Liberta, Lidwina, Margaret of Cortona, Margaret of Hungary, Ontcommer (or Uncumber), and Wilgefortis. One of the few male saints included in this list is Swiss hermit Nicholas of Flüe.

1347   Birthdate of Caterina di Giacomo di Benincasa, later to become Saint Catherine, a famous example of a life of self-starvation.

1554   German physician Johannes Lange publishes his Book *Medicinalium Epistolarum Miscellanea* (*Miscellaneous Medical Letters*), in which he describes a condition that he calls *morbus virgineus* ("virgin's disease") because it occurs only among virgins. The disease has a number of distinctive characteristics, one of which involves the skin's developing a greenish tint. This property leads to the name by which it was then known for another three centuries, the "greensickness." Lange recommended that an afflicted woman copulate with a man, which would then cure her disease. The disease has also been known as *chlorosis*, for the Greek term for "green." The condition today is known as hypochromic anemia and is not associated with a person's sexual experience.

1563   In his book, *An Excellent Treatise of Wounds Made with Gonneshot*, English surgeon Thomas Gale describes a condition now known as *geophasia* (the eating of earthy materials). The condition is a subset of the eating disorder known as pica. Although the condition was well known and frequently described during classical times, Gale's book is probably the first technical description of geophasia or pica.

1599   One of the best-known examples of the "miraculous maids" of the Middle Ages was Eva Fleigen (or Flegen or Fliegen), of Meurs (Germany). Reports tell of her refusal to eat throughout most of her life and her life having been endangered on one occasion by having eaten a single cherry and on a second occasion by having taken a spoonful of chicken soup.

Seventeenth and eighteenth centuries   The practice of self-starvation becomes more widespread among nonclerical, primarily young, women who adopt the practice for a variety of both sacred and secular reasons. The women are referred to, in general, as the *miraculous maids* or *miraculous maidens*.

1618   Italian anatomist Hieronymus Fabricius (also known as Girolamo Fabrizio, Fabricus ab Aquapendente, and Girolamo Fabrizi) describes two cases of rumination disorder in patients with hiatal hernia. Although the disorder had been known as far back as classical Greece, Fabricius's research was probably the first modern report on the condition. (An autopsy of one patient showed that he had a single stomach, in contrast with prevailing beliefs at the time that a person with rumination disorder would have at least two stomachs, similar to ruminating mammals.)

1669   English physician John Reynolds offers a paper to the Royal Society on "A Discourse upon Prodigious Abstinence," the "famed Derbyshire damosell," who survived for 12 months on "a few drops of the Syrup of stew'd Prunes, Water and Sugar, or the juice of a roasted Raisin, &c." The purpose of the paper was that such an event could occur without any form of miraculous intervention but as the result of bodily changes that adapt a person to such meager food intake (text available at http://quod.lib.umich.edu/e/eebo/A57186.0001.001?rgn=main;view=fulltext).

1679   Swiss physician Théophile Bonet publishes his book *Sepulchretum*, reporting on his dissection of obese individuals, the first such written record in Western history.

1685   Swiss anatomist Johannes (John) Conrad Peyer publishes the first truly scientific discussion of ruminant disorder in his book *Merycologia sive de Ruminantibus et Ruminatione Commentarius* (*Commentary on Ruminants and Domestic Ruminants*). Although the condition had been mentioned earlier in history (*see* **1618**), Peyer's description was a more detailed report on nine cases of merycism (rumination disorder).

1694 In an English translation of his book in Latin, *Phthisiologia* (1689), English physician Richard Morton describes a condition that he calls *nervous atrophy* or *nervous consumption* that appears to be anorexia nervosa. He describes the disease as "a wasting of Body without any remarkable Fever, Cough, or Shortness of Breath; but it is attended with a want of Appetite, and a bad digestion, upon which there follows a Languishing Weakness of Nature, and a falling away of the Flesh every day more and more."

1727 English physician Thomas Short publishes the first-known treatise on obesity, entitled *A Discourse Concerning the Causes and Effects of Corpulency: Together with the Method for Its Prevention and Cure*.

1727 Orsola Giuliani (later, Saint Victoria) dies, at least in part because of her long practice of anorexia. The interesting point about her life is that she was also known to engage in periods of episodes that might be classified today as binge eating and bulimia, when she supposedly was tempted by Satan and "ate everything in sight."

1780 English physician William Cullen describes obesity ("excessive corpulence") as a type of disease in his *Synopsis of Nosology*, a new system for classifying diseases. He claims that the decision results from an "increase of oil in the cellular texture of the body."

ca. nineteenth century Geophagia is common among slaves from Africa in South and North America, especially the American South. The practice has been so common among this population that even until relatively recently, bags of earth were sold to African Americans at bus stops in the South. At one point, the condition was so widespread and so harmful to a slave's work that some plantation owners fitted their slaves with masks that prevented them from eating without release from the masks.

1813   One of the best-known falsifications in the history of self-starvation is revealed in the case of Ann Moore, of Tutbury, Staffordshire, England. Moore had reached a condition of abject poverty in the early 1800s, at which point she announced that she was unable to eat food or drink. A number of investigations were conducted to validate her claim, all of which found no indication of falsehood. She earned a substantial amount of money from individuals who wished to visit and observe her, eventually depositing a total of £400 in 1812, apparently earned from such activities. A year later, her perfidy was revealed, and she died shortly thereafter.

1825   The French lawyer, politician, and gourmand Jean Anthelme Brillat-Savarin publishes an influential textbook *The Physiology of Taste*, in which he recommends what is probably the world's earliest low-carbohydrate diet. The diet is based on his philosophy that one of the primary causes of obesity is "the floury and starchy substances which man makes the prime ingredients of his daily nourishment. As we have said already, all animals that live on farinaceous food grow fat willy-nilly; and man is no exception to the universal law."

1835   In his classic work on social physics, *Sur L'homme et Le Développement De Ses Facultés, Ou Essai De Physique Sociale* (*On Man and the Development of His Faculties, or Essays on Social Physics*), Belgian polymath Adolphe Quetelet describes the body mass index (BMI), which eventually became the standard way of measuring a person's normal weight, underweight, or overweight.

1844   Mauritian physiologist Charles-Édouard Brown-Séquard develops a case of rumination disorder as a result of his own experiments on the contents of the human stomach. In his research, Brown-Séquard swallowed and then extracted a small sponge, the composition of which then revealed the contents of his stomach. After completing the experiment, he found that he was unable to break his habit of regurgitating and then once more swallowing his food.

1849   In his classic paper "Observations on the Development of the Fat Vesicle," British physician and microscopist Arthur Hill Hassall first describes the structure and development of fat cells.

1859   American psychiatrist William Stout Chipley describes a condition observed in mental hospitals characterized by an individual's refusal to eat. Chipley notes that the condition is caused by one of two factors: religious visions that warn against the consumption of food or an irrational fear of food. Chipley's observations are largely ignored by the wider psychiatric community and eventually held to have no connection with anorexia.

1860   French psychiatrist Louis-Victor Marcé publishes a paper "Note sur une forme de délire hypocondriaque consécutive aux dyspepsies et caractérisée principalement par le refus d'aliments" ("On a Form of Hypochondriacal Delirium Occurring Consecutive to Dyspepsia and Characterized by Refusal of Food") that appears to be the first written description of an eating disorder as a type of mental disorder. Marcé draws attention, in particular, to the obstinacy with which anorexics maintain their program of self-starvation. He insists that such individuals be removed from their homes because of the influence their families appear to have on their condition.

1863   An English carpenter and undertaker, William Banting, writes what is generally recognized as the first book on dieting, *Letter on Corpulence Addressed to the Public*. Banting's diet roughly corresponds to the "low-carbohydrate" diets still popular today that avoid sugary and starchy foods.

1868   English physician William Gull describes "a peculiar form of disease occurring mostly in young women, and characterised by extreme emaciation," one of the earliest scientific descriptions of anorexia nervosa. Gull calls the condition *apepsia hysteria*, although the name is later changed, first, to *anorexia hysterica* and later to its present name. (Also see 1873.)

1869   A 12-year-old Welsh girl by the name of Sarah Jacobs dies of self-starvation after a period of observation by nurses from Guy's Hospital to confirm that she actually was receiving no food or water. About two weeks after the observation began, she died from starvation. Her death was the subject of great interest throughout the nation and is thought to have inspired other girls to engage in the same activity.

1873   Gull (*see* **1868**) publishes a paper in the journal *Obesity Research* on his 1868 lecture on anorexia nervosa. (The full text of the paper is available at http://onlinelibrary.wiley.com/doi/10.1002/j.1550-8528.1997.tb00677.x/pdf.) In the same year, French physician Charles Lasègue publishes a similar paper on the topic of anorexia. The close proximity of the two papers raises questions as to which researcher deserves credit for first describing the disorder, a dispute that has yet to be fully resolved. (The full version of this paper can be found at http://onlinelibrary.wiley.com/doi/10.1002/j.1550-8528.1997.tb00676.x/epdf.)

1903   French psychologist Pierre Janet provides an anecdotal description of a condition that was probably bulimia. His patient, Nadja, had been obsessed by her body image since the age of four, and, as an adult, she limited herself to two helpings of clear soup, one egg yolk, a teaspoon of vinegar, and one cup of very strong tea each day. Janet's diagnosis was anorexia, although most authorities today feel that Nadja's case was probably more like the modern definition of bulimia.

1914   German pathologist Morris Simmonds describes a patient with lesions of the pituitary gland, who demonstrated the characteristics of anorexia nervosa. This, and additional reports of the same phenomenon in other autopsies, leads some authorities to believe that the condition of hypopituitarism is the (or a) cause of anorexia, leading to the much greater use of hormones to treat the condition.

1916   Mollie Fancher, widely known as the "Brooklyn Enigma," dies in New York City. She achieved considerable fame during her life because of her claims that she could go many weeks or months without eating, claims that were never confirmed by independent observers.

1922 Bohemia writer Franz Kafka publishes a short story called "Ein Hungerkünstler" ("A Hunger Artist"). The story tells of a man representing a pattern of self-starvation at the time, carried out entirely by males. These "performers" appeared in sideshows, circuses, and other popular forms of entertainment. Their "act" was the intentional avoidance of food for periods of up to 40 days (after which audiences were said to have tired of the performance). The occupation was lucrative to those who took part in the practice.

1936 English physician John A. Ryle publishes an article, "Anorexia Nervosa," in *The Lancet*, in which he makes a strong argument that anorexia is a mental and psychological problem and not an organic malfunction. He says at one point in treating patients that "the absence of 'organic disease' must be confidently stressed." Ryle's paper, followed shortly by a series of similar articles, reflects the abandonment of endocrinological explanations for the occurrence of anorexia.

1940 Stanford University psychiatrist Regina C. Casper publishes an article, "On the Emergence of Bulimia Nervosa as a Syndrome: A Historical View," in which she attempts to trace the occurrence of a bulimia-like eating disorder throughout recorded history. The conclusion is that the condition is exceedingly rare until the early 1940s, when reports of bulimia begin to appear more frequently in the professional literature.

1945 German psychiatrist Ludwig Binswanger publishes one of the most famous papers in the history of psychiatry and the history of eating disorders, "Der Fall Ellen West" ("The Case of Ellen West"). The paper describes an American woman, Ellen West, who suffered from anorexia throughout her adolescence and adult life. Binswanger attempted to use a new type of psychoanalysis to treat West but eventually decided she could not be helped. She viewed death as the only way of escaping her problem and all but starved herself to death for most of her adult life. She finally died in 1921 by committing suicide with poison.

1952   Anorexia is listed for the first time in the *Diagnostic and Statistical Manual of Mental Disorders (DSM-I)* as a psychophysiological disorder, a psychophysiological order in which some behavioral characteristic(s) can be explained by biological (physiological) factors.

1955   American psychiatrist Albert Stunkard provides the first description of a condition that he calls *night-eating syndrome.*

1959   Stunkard (**1955**) provides the first scientific explanation of the condition now known as *binge eating disorder.*

1967   University of Michigan sociologist Richard B. Stuart describes the use of behavioral therapy for the treatment of obesity.

1968   University of Iowa surgeons Edward E. Mason and Chikashi Ito describe the first use of gastric bypass surgery as a method of treating obesity.

1978   Two surgeons in New Mexico, Lawrence H. Wilkinson and Ole A. Peloso, develop a method known as bariatric surgery for the treatment of gross obesity.

1979   British psychologist Gerald Russell provides the first scientific description of an anorexia-like disorder that he calls bulimia nervosa. The paper, "Bulimia Nervosa: An Ominous Variant of Anorexia Nervosa," appears in the journal *Psychological Medicine.*

1980   Eating disorders for the first time receive a separate and distinct entry in the *DSM-III* as a mental disorder. Bulimia nervosa is also listed in *DSM-III* for the first time.

1980   A category called *atypical eating disorders* is included for the first time in *DSM-III*. The disorder is vaguely classified as any type of eating disorder that cannot otherwise be described as anorexia nervosa, bulimia nervosa, or pica. In the revision of

DSM-III, called *DSM-IIIR* (1987), the name was changed to eating disorder not otherwise specified in *DSM-IV* and again to other specified feeding or eating disorder in *DSM-V*.

1984   *Glamour* magazine conducts a survey of 33,000 women, asking how they feel about their bodies. Forty-one percent of respondents say they are unhappy with their bodies, and about 75 percent say they are "too fat." Actual physical measurements provided for the sample indicate that only about 25 percent are actually overweight. A similar survey conducted by *Vogue* magazine in 1986 finds that about 70 percent of fourth-grade girls are concerned about their weight and about half have started some type of dieting program. (*Also see* **2014**.)

1985   Italian psychiatrist Mara Selvini Palazzoli publishes an article, "Anorexia Nervosa: A Syndrome of the Affluent Society," in which she makes the argument that anorexia is a cultural phenomenon. She uses as an example the total absence of anorexia cases in Italy during World War II (1939–1945), which she attributes to food shortages at the time, followed by a flood of such cases in the years immediately following the end of the war, during which the Italian economy blossomed and a surplus of food became readily available (*Transcultural Psychiatry*. 22(3): 199–205).

1986   *See* **1984**.

1987   Rumination disorder is listed for the first time in the *DSM-III*.

Late 1990s   Pro-anorexia websites begin showing up on the Internet. The purpose of the websites is to promote the practice of anorexia and bulimia, especially among younger women. The sites are also known as pro-ana (for anorexia) and pro-mia (for bulimia) websites. Although strongly opposed by medical and eating disorder groups, the websites have continued to thrive into the late 2010s.

1994   Eating disorders not otherwise specified (EDNOS) is listed in the *Diagnostic and Statistical Manual of Mental Disorders* (*DSM-IV*) for the first time.

1996   California physician Steven Bratman suggests the existence of a type of eating disorder that he calls *orthorexia* ("correct appetite"), in which individuals strive to achieve what they view as the healthiest possible diet but which may have harmful nutritional effects.

1997   A report issued by the World Health Organization, "Obesity: Preventing and Managing the Global Epidemic," establishes a system for identifying various types of obesity and explains how it has become a worldwide issue of epidemic proportions.

1999   The state of California passes the Mental Health Parity Act, the first law of its kind requiring health insurers to provide the same level of mental health care (including treatment for eating disorders) as they do for physical health problems. (*Also see* **2008** and **2015**.)

2000   In the case of *Frank v. United Airlines*, the Ninth Circuit Court of Appeals rules that plaintiffs ("Frank"), a group of flight attendants, had not shown that the airline's weight restrictions had been responsible for the eating disorders they developed as a result of trying to meet that policy. The court also ruled that having different weight standards for men and women was unconstitutional.

2002   A team of researchers at the University of Pittsburgh report the first discovery of a possible genetic cause for anorexia. They find a mutation at locus D1S3721 at chromosome site 1p34.2 as the possible culprit for the development of anorexia.

2006   The Italian government adopts a voluntary "anti-anorexia" code designed to deal with the nation's problem of "ultrathin" models. Model agencies and related companies may choose to sign or not sign the code, without penalty for the latter choice.

2008   The Binge Eating Disorder Association is founded.

2008   The U.S. Congress passes the Paul Wellstone and Pete Domenici Mental Health Parity and Addiction Equity Act of 2008, requiring that group health plans and health insurance issuers provide mental health or substance use disorder benefits equivalent to those for medical and surgical benefits.

2010   The Spanish legislature passes a law banning advertisements that promote products and treatments designed to help someone have a "perfect body."

2010   The legislature of the state of New York adopts new legislation design to protect individuals under the age of 18 from being forced or encouraged to meet weight standards when they are employed in certain lines of work, such as modeling and stage, television, and film work.

2010s   Eating disorders begin to appear more commonly in popular films and television shows, such as the Netflix special *To the Bone* (2017). The programs elicit a storm of controversy over the portrayal of eating disorders, suggesting, to some observers, that they have positive value for teenage women, a charge that other critics reject.

2011   The Ninth Circuit Court of Appeals rules in *Harlick v. Blue Shield of California* that the plaintiff is entitled to payment for treatment for her anorexia nervosa disorder, not because it was specifically required in her Blue Cross health insurance plan but because the state of California's Mental Health Parity Act does so.

2013   An Israeli law designed to control eating disorders in models and certain other performers goes into effect. Among the law's provision is a requirement that such individuals have a BMI of at least 18.5. "Photoshopping" of photographs to encourage efforts to reach an "ideal weight" is also prohibited.

2013   The Center of Excellence for Eating Disorders at the University of North Carolina announces the beginning of the Anorexia Nervosa Genetics Initiative (ANGI), a program designed to detect genetic variations that may be responsible for the development of eating disorders.

2014   *Glamour* magazine conducts a follow-up of its 1984 study (q.v.) on women's perception of their own body image. The survey finds that the fraction of respondents who are "unhappy with their body" has actually increased over the 30-year period, from 41 percent in 1948 to 54 percent in 2014. In addition, 80 percent of respondents said that "looking in a mirror" makes them feel unhappy.

2015   The U.S. Food and Drug Administration (FDA) approves the use of lisdexamfetamine dimesylate (Vyvanse) for the treatment of binge eating disorder. The drug was originally developed for the treatment of attention deficit hyperactivity disorder but was then found to be helpful in dealing with binge eating disorder also.

2015   Missouri becomes the first state to pass a law specifically requiring insurance companies to pay for all "medically necessary" treatment for eating disorders.

2015   India's Supreme Court rules that members of the Jain religion may continue their traditional practice of fasting as a way of committing suicide. (*Also see* **sixth century** BCE.)

2016   The U.S. Congress adopts the 21st Century Cures Act. Among its many provisions is legislation dealing with federal financial support for research on and education about eating disorders. Those provisions were included in an early bill passed by the House of Representatives, the Helping Families in Mental Health Crisis Act of 2016.

2017   The French legislature approves a law designed to protect individuals from eating disorders by banning weight standards to which models must adhere.

Glossary

Discussions of eating disorders often involve terminology that is unfamiliar to the average person. In some cases, the terms are scientific or medical expressions used most commonly by professionals in the field. In other cases, the terms may be part of the everyday vernacular that some people may *think* they understand, but that actually have more precise meanings. This glossary defines some of those terms that have been used in this book, along with some other terms that one may encounter in additional research on the topic.

amenorrhea   The loss of menstrual periods for a period of at least three months.

animal therapy   A system of treatment that uses dogs, cats, and other animals to facilitate a person's ability to understand and deal with his or her eating disorder issues.

anxiety disorder   An excessive sense of anxiety and worry that persists for at least a few months and that interferes with a person's ability to accomplish daily tasks.

art therapy   (also known as expressive arts or creative arts therapy) A method of treating eating disorders that makes use of the fine arts, music, dramatics, role-playing, storytelling, movement, writing, or other forms of expression as a way of dealing with the issues that may lie at the heart of an eating disorder.

body checking   A pattern of thoughts and/or behaviors induced by a person's concern about his or her physical appearance.

body dysmorphic disorder   A person's belief that his or her body is severely flawed in some way or another, such as being too fat or not muscular enough.

body image   The perception that a person has about his or her body, which may or may not correspond with the perception of a neutral observer.

bradycardia   An abnormally slow heart rate of usually less than about 60 beats per minute.

cognitive behavioral therapy   A widely used method for treating mental disorders in which a therapist helps a patient to understand the basis for his or her disorder and to develop methods for dealing with that disorder.

dialectical behavioral therapy   A treatment method originally developed for borderline personality disorder, focusing on skill development in four areas: distress tolerance, emotion, interpersonal skills, and regulation of emotions.

differential diagnosis   The process of identifying one specific disease or disorder, rather than some other disease or disorder, as being most likely the cause of a person's health problems.

edema   The swelling of some part of the body because of the accumulation of liquids.

emesis   The act of vomiting.

emetic   A substance that will induce vomiting.

enema   A method used to induce defecation by the injection of a liquid or gaseous material into the rectum.

epidemiology   The science that deals with the incidence, prevalence, spread, and possible control of a disease.

etiology   The study of the cause(s) of a disease or other physical or mental condition.

forbidden foods   Foods that a person regards as being "off limits," for one reason or another, and are therefore excluded from his or her diet.

functional dysphagia   The inability or unwillingness to swallow all or some types of food.

hypoglycemia   Low blood sugar.

hypokalemia   Low levels of potassium in the blood.

hyponatremia   Low levels of sodium in the blood.

incidence   The number of new cases of a disease or condition over some given period of time, such as one month or one year.

ketosis   A medical condition that develops when the body ingests an inadequate amount of carbohydrates and begins to metabolize fats. The condition has serious, some fatal, consequences.

lanugo   A fine, downy hair that grows on the body after a prolonged period of inadequate food intake.

lapse   The occurrence of a single failure in a person's attempt to overcome some condition, such as anorexia or bulimia (*also see* **relapse**).

medication management   The use of certain types of drugs to control an eating disorder, such as antidepressants, antiepileptics, antiobesity, and antiaddiction drugs, or drugs used against attention deficit hyperactivity disorder.

morbidity   The condition of having a disease.

orthorexia   A term not yet officially accepted by most specialists in the field of eating disorders that describes a condition in which a person's diet is controlled by the selection of only certain types of "healthy" foods.

osteopenia   Bone density that is lower than normal but not low enough to be diagnosed as osteoporosis.

osteoporosis   A condition in which a person's bones become weak and brittle, with a density significantly less than that expected for his or her age and weight.

PEG tube   (percutaneous endoscopic gastrostomy tube) A tube that is surgically implanted into a person's stomach through the abdomen. It is used to deliver liquid nutrition to the digestive system for a person who is not obtaining those nutrients through a normal diet.

perfectionism   An attitude that some aspect of a person's life must be without flaw, such as having an ideal ("perfect") body size and shape.

prevalence   The number of individuals who have a given disease or disorder in a population over some given period of time, such as one month or one year.

psychoeducation   The process of providing information and/ or instruction to an individual as a way of treating his or her mental disorder.

purging   The process of intentionally eliminating materials from the body, through either the mouth (emesis) or the rectum (defecation).

relapse   The resumption of some condition from which one is attempting to recover, such as an eating disorder.

risk factor   Any condition or situation that increases the likelihood that a person will develop a disease or disorder.

sign   An indication of a person's lack of well-being that can be detected by an outside observer. A temperature reading is a sign.

subthreshold disorder   A condition in which a person displays all or some of the signs and symptoms of a medical disorder and that interferes with a person's normal life but is not yet serious enough to be formally diagnosed for that condition.

symptom   An indication of a person's disease state based on reports that he or she provides to someone but that cannot be detected directly by that outside person. A headache is a symptom.

syncope   A temporary loss of consciousness caused by an insufficiency of oxygen in the brain, often the result of low blood sugar or low blood pressure.

tachycardia   A rapid resting pulse rate, generally defined as 100 beats per minute or more.

Index

Note: Page numbers followed by *t* indicate tables.

About the Author

David E. Newton holds an associate's degree in science from Grand Rapids (Michigan) Junior College, a BA in chemistry (with high distinction), an MA in education from the University of Michigan, and an EdD in science education from Harvard University. He is the author of more than 400 textbooks, encyclopedias, resource books, research manuals, laboratory manuals, trade books, and other educational materials. He taught mathematics, chemistry, and physical science in Grand Rapids, Michigan, for 13 years; was professor of chemistry and physics at Salem State College in Massachusetts for 15 years; and was adjunct professor in the College of Professional Studies at the University of San Francisco for 10 years.

The author's previous books for ABC-CLIO include *Global Warming* (1993), *Gay and Lesbian Rights—A Resource Handbook* (1994, 2009), *The Ozone Dilemma* (1995), *Environmental Justice* (1996, 2009), *Violence and the Mass Media* (1996), *Encyclopedia of Cryptology* (1997), *Social Issues in Science and Technology: An Encyclopedia* (1999), *DNA Technology* (2009, 2016), *Sexual Health* (2010), *Same-Sex Marriage* (2011, 2016), *The Animal Experimentation Debate* (2013), *Marijuana* (2013, 2017), *World Energy Crisis* (2013), *GMO Food* (2014), *Science and Political Controversy* (2014), *Steroids and Doping in Sports* (2014, 2018), *Fracking* (2015), *Solar Energy* (2015), *Wind Energy* (2015), *Global Water Crisis* (2016), *Youth Drug Abuse* (2016), *Youth Substance Abuse* (2016), *Sex and Gender* (2017), and *Sexually Transmitted Diseases* (2018). His other recent books include *Physics: Oryx Frontiers of Science Series* (2000); *Sick!*

(four volumes) (2000); *Science, Technology, and Society: The Impact of Science in the 19th Century* (two volumes, 2001); *Encyclopedia of Fire* (2002); *Molecular Nanotechnology: Oryx Frontiers of Science Series* (2002); *Encyclopedia of Water* (2003); *Encyclopedia of Air* (2004); *Nuclear Power* (2005); *Stem Cell Research* (2006); *Latinos in the Sciences, Math, and Professions* (2007); *The New Chemistry* (six volumes, 2007); and *DNA Evidence and Forensic Science* (2008). He has also been an updating and consulting editor on a number of books and reference works, including *Chemical Compounds* (2005); *Chemical Elements* (2006); *Encyclopedia of Endangered Species* (2006); *World of Chemistry* (2006); *World of Health* (2006); *World of Mathematics* (2006); *UXL Encyclopedia of Science* (2007); *Alternative Medicine* (2008); *Community Health* (2009); *Genetic Medicine* (2009); *Grzimek's Animal Life Encyclopedia* (2009); *The Gale Encyclopedia of Medicine* (2010–2011); *The Gale Encyclopedia of Alternative Medicine* (2013); *Discoveries in Modern Science: Exploration, Invention, and Technology* (2013–2014); and *Science in Context* (2013–2014).